D1157604

WHAT
SHOULD
I DO?

Kirk House Publishers

WHAT SHOULD I DO?

A FAMILY PHYSICIAN
DISCUSSES ABORTION,
RELIGIOUS FREEDOM, AND
DIFFICULT DECISIONS

Jeffrey D. Nelson, M.D.

Paperback ISBN: 978-1-952976-36-0
LCCN: 2021923444

Cover and interior design by Ann Aubitz

First Printing: November 2021
First Edition

Published by Kirk House Publishers
1250 E 115th Street
Burnsville, MN 55337
Kirkhousepublishers.com
612-781-2815

Foreword

Until my junior year in high school, abortion was largely a theoretical issue left for debate in social studies class. But then I heard that a recent graduate who had been drafted sent his former girlfriend a coat hanger when she told him that she was pregnant. Suddenly, when I knew both people involved, this issue took on new significance. It was 1971, before *Roe v. Wade*. It was a time when we talked in hushed tones about girls getting "back-alley abortions" or traveling to New York, where abortion was legal. Now it was real.

Ever since then—as a man, husband, father, pastor, and citizen—I have struggled with the real-life implications of our human sexuality in all its forms. So has Dr. Jeff Nelson, as a fine medical doctor, husband, father, citizen, and follower of Jesus. I appreciate the seriousness with which Dr. Nelson has dealt with abortion, and the helpful, humble case he has made in this book. There are plenty of voices that claim to speak for God these days. As a pastor, I am familiar with that dynamic. But Dr. Nelson has clearly laid out his argument for a "pro-choice/ pro-life" position on abortion. It is mine as well. And I believe that it is a faithful, godly position to hold. I want abortion to be safe, legal, and rare—available to girls like my 1971 acquaintance who was sent the metal coat hanger as an encouragement to end her pregnancy herself.

Of course, wading into these waters will stir up all sorts of pushback. Dr. Nelson courageously takes on this task—and I appreciate it. I trust that those who want to learn more about the dynamics involved in this contro-versial issue will find this book to be helpful, as I did.

May God bless us all as we struggle for clarity and harmony.

Pastor Rolf E. Olson
St. Paul, Minnesota
B.A., St. Olaf College
Master of Divinity, Luther Theological Seminary

Meet the Author

Who am I? I believe I am a child of God, created and sustained by the wonderful loving and grace-filled entity that created this universe and the human species in it and nourishes us every day.

I was born to parents of Swedish descent in a Midwestern town in Iowa, raised in a Lutheran church, attended Luther College in Decorah, Iowa, and then went to medical school at the University of Iowa. I met the love of my life at Luther and married her the summer before I started medical school. Jane was the most wonderful and amazing part of my life, but sadly she died in 2016 from a primary brain cancer. I firmly believe God created her, loved her, and sustained both of us through the terribly difficult time of her cancer. I believe her soul exists in the heavenly realm with God. I am so blessed to have shared so much time with her, my children, and the rest of my family. Life should be valued as precious for each one of us.

Jane wanted me to find another woman to live with after she died. She did not think I would do well living by myself for the rest of my life. I could not think of such things when she was alive. Time does heal some wounds, to some extent. I wrote a book about Jane, *I Got to Live With an Angel*.

I did not expect I would be blessed again with a loving relationship with another wonderful woman, Libby. She had to experience the tragedy of the death of her son from brain cancer when he was only eight years old. I cannot imagine the death of one of my children. I had patients in my practice who lost children. I had patients who had children with life-threatening illnesses, such as acute leukemia. Whether it was recent or a long time ago, my patients who had experienced childhood death had a scar that never fully healed. The death of a child can often be the death of a family—Libby's marriage ended in divorce before we met. I am so sorry she had to endure those painful events in her life. While I wish she did not have to experience this, I am so thankful for her love in my life. We are both physicians, and the tragedies we have seen in our patients as well as the tragedies in our personal lives have molded us to be who we are today.

After medical school, I went through residency at the St. Paul Ramsey Family Practice program in St. Paul, Minnesota, from 1979 to 1982. I worked harder the first two years of this program than I ever have in my life. One week, while on the Newborn Intensive Care Unit, I worked 126 hours, which does not leave many hours to eat or sleep. This was before the number of hours worked per week was limited by residency programs. We routinely worked 80 hours per week, but it was often up to 90–100 hours per week. After being on call in the hospital, and usually being up most of the night, and working the following day—I would go home and fall asleep eating dinner with my wife. I was not such a great companion then!

St. Paul Ramsey Hospital subsequently became Regions Hospital in St. Paul when the HMO HealthPartners bought the hospital. Their residency program was closed in 2006. Things begin and things end—which is the case in all of life.

Table of Contents

Chapter 1: Setting Guidelines

As a family medicine physician, I worked at the same clinic and in the same community of Cottage Grove, Minnesota, from the summer of 1982 until I retired from practice in 2020. I did obstetrics for about 18 of those years and delivered numerous babies. Whenever my partners and I were not out of town on vacation, we delivered our own obstetrical patients even if we were not on call for the rest of our group. Deliveries nearly always happened at night, on weekends, or in the evenings. Only occasionally were we called out of the daytime office schedule for a delivery. Several of my partners stopped doing OB in the 1990s, and it was around the year 2000 when I decided to free up more time for my family by not delivering any more babies.

While I was doing OB, many of my patients had unplanned pregnancies. Some of them carried their pregnancy to term and had a child. Some of those children were placed for adoption. Some of those children were kept by their mother. Some of the women decided it was best to have an abortion for many different reasons.

I am a white male. You might ask how I can understand and write about women with unintended pregnancies. True, I cannot fully understand what I have not experienced myself. I can only share my thoughts, my experiences, and some of the experiences of those I have met in my life. I ask you, the reader, to imagine you are the woman dealing with each situation I present in this book. We need to try to understand how another person is feeling and thinking.

From both my professional and personal experience, my wishes for the readers of this book are that:

✓ As many people as possible understand *the reality of contraception and abortion and pregnancy*. It would be helpful if most people in our society tried to follow the science and not the falsehoods that are promoted.

✓ The readers understand how *freedom of religion* in our country requires that both contraception and abortion be easily available for those who wish to use these health care services.

✓ The readers understand the risks that *a woman takes when she becomes pregnant* and that a woman views those risks very differently when she desires to become pregnant, as compared to when she must deal with an unintended pregnancy.

✓ "Pro-life" people understand that freedom of religion requires them *to not force their beliefs on the rest of the population.*

- ✓ "Pro-choice" people *understand the challenge* the above represents for a "pro-life" person.
- ✓ More people *become "pro-choice/pro-life"*—as I am trying to explain it in my book.

As I walk my faith journey, I continue to realize how each one of us is buffeted in life by many challenges.

The apostle Paul writes in the Bible in the book of Galatians 5:19-21 the following: "The acts of the sinful nature are obvious: sexual immorality, impurity and debauchery; idolatry and witchcraft; hatred, discord, jealousy, fits of rage, selfish ambition, dissensions, factions and envy; drunkenness, orgies, and the like."

That is followed by one of my favorite verses, Galatians 5:22: "But the fruit of the Spirit is love, joy, peace, patience, kindness, goodness, faithfulness, gentleness and self-control." God loves all of us the same—I believe that is one of the main messages God has for us.

None of us are perfect. I hope and pray that all people get to experience God's love as I have been blessed to experience it in my life so far. God's grace and love are infinite, which is so difficult for us all to understand.

I believe no matter who we are, we have more to learn in our lives.

I ask all of us to try to be more considerate of others in our society—and to try to better understand what the other is thinking. I ask all of us to try to "Love thy neighbor as thyself." This book covers a heavy subject. It is okay to read a chapter or two at a time—and then think about it. As you ponder, I ask you to consider how you would feel if your beliefs were different.

I pray that God's spirit fills me and guides me as I try to express these thoughts, which I believe God wants me to share for your consideration. Whether you currently consider yourself to be "pro-choice," "pro-life," or "I don't know," I hope you will find my thoughts useful to consider.

I am trying to share some of the thoughts a woman may have when dealing with an unplanned pregnancy. Each woman has a different set of beliefs and life experiences that lead her to different conclusions about what is best to do. When asked, "Doctor, should I do it?" I could not respond yes or no. I needed to help the woman consider what she believed, what she felt her options were, and what the pros and cons were for her in this situation. In all of healthcare, *the patient has the right to decide what will happen to their body.*

Chapter 2: My Ideal World

In my ideal world, a man and a woman would fall in love and get married before having intercourse. Each would be open and honest about how they feel—and be able to express their desires for their relationship. Each would be able to respond in a healthy fashion to those feelings and desires. Neither would desire to control or harm the other, which would be because their love for each other was pure and perfect. When they desired to have children, their intercourse would result in a pregnancy in which both the mother and the fetus were healthy and had no complications. The labor and delivery would be uncomplicated, and the result would be a healthy newborn baby both parents loved. Either parent could be any racial or ethnic background, and throughout their lives they would continue to learn from each other. They would teach their child to love and learn as they had loved and learned. Those parents would remain married and healthy until they grew old, and their child would be able to become an adult before either of them died.

In that *ideal world*, there would be no need for abortion.

I have yet to see anyone who has actually been able to live in that ideal world. My parents divorced when I was 29 years old. I was happily married and had two children then, but it was still a difficult time. I was thankful it did not happen when I was younger. My mom wanted me to pick her side and blame my dad for the divorce. She could not see the role she played. I think her lack of self-confidence prevented her from accepting any responsibility in the divorce. I loved both of my parents, and I could not choose sides.

My wife died after we had been married for 41 years. She was able to see the birth of two of our grandchildren. I now have six grandchildren, and I know she would have loved to be a part of their lives. I know she would have loved to continue to be a part of the lives of our children—and I know how much that would have meant to them. But apparently, *some things are not meant to be.*

Sometimes, we love another person, but they do not love us back. Sometimes, a man and a woman love each other, but tragedy strikes one of them unexpectedly. Many times, intimacy and sexual intercourse occur prior to marriage. Even if contraception is used, it is not perfect—and pregnancy before marriage is not rare.

I do remember how Jane and I were hoping we would not have to deal with an unintended pregnancy. When we were in college, and when we were married and I was in medical school, we were not ready to be parents. It was not long after our relationship became serious that Jane started to use the birth control pill.

Some of us simply live a significant part of our life before finding the one special person we love. There are many reasons why the world is not an ideal world. But we always must do the best that we can. Each one of us must make the most of the world we are given.

I describe my *practical* world in Chapter 16.

The sexual issues of those who are lesbian, gay, bisexual, or transgender are beyond the scope of this book. I consider these persons to be equal to any other human being. I have had the honor to meet or know some amazing individuals who are in those categories. They are not included in this discussion simply because they are not the majority of the human population—and a human pregnancy requires male sperm and a female egg, as well as a functioning uterus, for the traditional process of pregnancy to occur. However, a gay couple using a surrogate mother to have a child, or a lesbian couple using artificial insemination, or either couple having a child through adoption, could have to deal with some of the complications of pregnancy I describe later.

As a family physician, I saw so many different situations. Some of them were caused by factors beyond the control of the individual patient. Some were factors where the patient could have chosen a different route for their life.

- I saw some patients who I believed made wise decisions—and some who made decisions that I thought were foolish.
- I saw women who wanted to be pregnant—but could not get pregnant.
- I saw women who did not want to be pregnant—but unfortunately had become pregnant.
- Some had used birth control, and it had failed.
- Some had intended to use birth control but did not.

So often, contraception has depended on only the efforts of the woman.

A man should be just as responsible as the woman for using effective contraception.

The main two options a man has for contraception currently are to use condoms or have a vasectomy when permanent contraception is desired. But a man can do more than that.

- He can understand and support the individual needs of the woman he has chosen to become intimate with.
- If he genuinely cares about this woman, he will make it clear to her that he will be responsible and caring.

- He will make it clear that if, as a couple, they decide to use a female form of contraception, he will help her as necessary to obtain and use it.
- He can let her know how he would feel if they were to have an unintended pregnancy.

Ideally, a couple would decide together how to manage this situation. But I do believe a man needs to respect what a woman would decide because she is the one who must handle the pregnancy and accept the risk to her health and her life.

In my ideal world, both the man and the woman would have the ability to control their impulse for procreation until they have effective contraception available—and then would use it consistently. But some individuals are very poor at stopping their actions based on an impulse. Some people have what is called an "impulse control disorder," where the person has much more difficulty than usual stopping an impulse. But I believe we all must be responsible for our actions, even if we have an impulse control disorder. At the same time, I believe we are all called to have compassion for someone who has suffered because of any of these situations.

At times, spontaneity can be a significant joy in life. The difference between spontaneity and an impulse that hurts another can be very narrow.

Because of the reality that our society still has a significant patriarchal bias, most contraception is still dependent on the woman's efforts. In my medical practice, some women had caring male partners, whether they were married or not. Some had male partners who did not seem to know the meaning of caring. Indeed, so many situations are experienced by people during their lifetimes.

Each one of us only knows our own experience. Whether through reading or talking with family and friends and others, we learn something about the experience of other people. But we can only imagine their experience—we truly only know our own experience. I hope that through the examples I will give later, you may have some insight into situations that you have not experienced. For any of you who have experienced the tragic circumstances I describe, I hope and pray you have had support from your family and friends.

There are some people who:

- Are sure they know what is best for another person to do.
- Are quick to tell another person what they should do in a particular situation.
- Are a little humbler than that.
- Will just listen to another and ask them what they think is best to do.

Each one of us is unique, and I do not believe there is any perfect combination of traits.

Chapter 3: Why Am I Writing This Book?

Why do I keep thinking about writing on the issues surrounding abortion? Is it my selfish desire to author a book? Is it God encouraging me to express my thoughts—or God's thoughts? Anyone reading this will come to his or her own conclusion. I don't know, but I do know my inner voice is encouraging me the more that I listen to it.

The biology of reproduction is a continuous cycle or circle of life in which the egg and sperm combine and form the fertilized egg, which replicates and undergoes differentiation and development through the embryo stage, the fetal stage, birth, and the development from an infant to a child to an adult. The adult may reproduce or not, and the cycle continues through the members of the species as long as this species exists.

The circle of your life is intertwined with the circles of those of your family, friends, and others you interact with. Our species is defined by the summation of all the circles of life—and how they are interconnected with each other. Each member of a species has DNA unique to this species. Each member also has DNA that is unique to that individual when the complexity of the DNA structure is at the level of our genus (a biological classification) and species: *Homo sapiens*.

No two human beings think exactly alike. To me, that is part of the beauty of life, and it is also part of the challenge in life. Most Christians believe God gave men and women free will—the ability to decide what they think is best to do in each situation. Free will in the human is not necessarily the same as God's will.

Regarding the issue of abortion, there are so many viewpoints on what is right and what is wrong. Even within the various denominations of Christianity, very many different views exist on this issue.

Ask yourself:

- Why do some Christians feel the need to interpret the Bible literally? Why do some interpret the creation story literally? "In the beginning, God created the heavens and the earth" (Genesis 1:1 New International Version or NIV).

- Is God only magnificent and wonderful if the world is created instantly according to the timeframe of man? Through the sum of my life, I believe God has taught me that His creation is beautiful and magnificent, not because it happened instantly in my timeframe, but because of the beauty and complexity of the entire creation.

- Is creation of the universe by God any less wonderful if it occurred according to the sequence in the latest scientific theory? How fantastic is the order and complexity of our universe! As we continue to unravel some of the mysteries of our world, I am awed at the amazing nature of this universe. **If this is all by chance, then we won the biggest Powerball in all of history.**
- Why do some Christians feel the need to interpret Bible stories in a very literal fashion, while other Christians, who are just as faithful, interpret the same verses so differently?
- How does one respect the sanctity of all life, including that of each woman? How does one do that in a country with freedom of religion?

As one who considered majoring in math in college, I believe the probability of this world being created by God is greater than the probability of chance causing it to happen. Could there be a mathematical theorem that expresses this? My first inclination was to say "no," but then who knows where theoretical mathematicians will take us in the future.

"So, God created man in his own image,
in the image of God he created him;
male and female he created them."
(Genesis 1:27)

Chapter 4: Definitions

To consider a subject, or discuss a subject together, we need to have a vocabulary understood by all. Although the below may seem obvious to some of you, I feel it is important to review.

- *Abortion:* the termination of pregnancy, whether spontaneous or induced.
- *Spontaneous abortion* or *miscarriage*: the termination of pregnancy that results without being directly induced by the act of a human. Many known medical reasons exist for spontaneous abortions, be it genetic abnormalities that are not compatible with continuing life or factors in the female genital tract or hormone system that cause a lack of an adequate environment for the fertilized egg to grow.
- *Induced abortion:* the termination of pregnancy caused by either the ingestion of a substance or the performance of a procedure.
- *Safe abortion:* the performance of an induced abortion according to methods accepted by the

medical community as appropriate for the individual's specific stage of pregnancy and situation.

- *Unsafe abortion:* the performance of an induced abortion not done according to the above, often by someone who is not a trained and licensed medical individual.
- *"Pro-choice":* the ethical belief that a woman has the right to decide whether to remain pregnant when that occurs.
- *"Pro-life":* the ethical belief that, in some or all cases, the process of induced abortion is ethically wrong or illegal—or against God's will.
- *Fertilized egg:* the physical entity that is the result of the fusion of an egg and a sperm before any further cell division and duplication has occurred, i.e., the result of conception.
- *Embryo:* "an animal in the early stages of growth and differentiation that are characterized by cleavage, the laying down of fundamental tissues, and the formation of primitive organs and organ systems—*especially:* the developing human individual from the time of implantation to the end of the eighth week after conception" (Miriam-Webster Dictionary).
- *Fetus:* "an unborn…vertebrate especially after attaining the basic structural plan of its kind—*specifically*: a developing human from usually

two months after conception to birth" (Miriam-Webster Dictionary).

- *Trimester in pregnancy:* one-third of the pregnancy. The first trimester is generally from conception until the 12th–13th week. The second trimester is from then until about 27–28 weeks of gestation. The third trimester is from that time until delivery, which usually occurs at about 40 weeks of gestation.

- *Point of viability:* The point in a pregnancy where the fetus has a significant chance of surviving outside of the uterus. Even with all the current medical knowledge and access to the latest treatments, if delivery occurs prior to 22–24 weeks, survival is very unlikely to occur. It is likely for there to be some type of permanent adverse results from that level of prematurity. The closer a pregnant woman is to her due date, which is 40 weeks of gestation, the better the chance the delivered infant does well.

Case #1

Jane, a 26-year-old married woman, had a planned pregnancy. She was low risk for any complications, and she and her husband, who was training to be a family physician, looked forward to their first child. Her pregnancy was uncomplicated until the fetus was in the breach position in the last month of pregnancy—and any attempts to change the position to the normal vertex or head position were unsuccessful.

Having a breach delivery for the first vaginal delivery is a much higher risk of complication, especially for the infant. When it is breech, the butt is delivered first, followed by the body and finally the head. It is not uncommon for the head to get stuck because of the position, as well as the cervix not being fully dilated. During the time it can take to get the head delivered, the umbilical cord is compressed by the head and so no blood is able to flow as usual through the umbilical cord. Lack of oxygen to the infant can cause brain damage and other health problems.

So, it was decided that Jane would have a Caesarean section (C-section) when she went into labor. This was a standard recommendation in 1980 when this occurred—and still is a standard recommendation today. Her C-section was done by a skilled obstetrician, but during the procedure, her bladder was nicked, which the surgeon did not realize. Post-operatively, she was slow to recover and had constipation. She was discharged home on the seventh day.

Just two days later, in the middle of the night, her intuition told her to return to the hospital. She had not had a bowel movement, her abdomen was increasingly distended, and she had begun having visual hallucinations. She was frightened by the changes occurring and fearful of what it might mean both for her and for her young son. At the hospital, she was evaluated by Dr. Rob Lund, one of the family-medicine first-year residents. He determined that her abdominal cavity was full of fluid, which was urine leaking from the bladder. This was effectively causing kidney failure because all the material that the kidneys were excreting was being reabsorbed back into her system by her peritoneum—the lining of the abdominal cavity. Her serum potassium was 7, which is extremely high and put Jane at risk for severe cardiac dysrhythmia, which could cause death.

After paracentesis—draining of the abdominal fluid—and correction of her severe electrolyte abnormalities, she had surgery to repair the bladder laceration. With repair of the bladder, her kidney function returned to normal, she healed up, and she was determined to breastfeed her infant, even though these various events had reduced her milk supply. She had two additional pregnancies and had to have two more C-sections. In her second pregnancy, she attempted vaginal birth after having had the first delivery as a C-section (VBAC). But her cervix did not dilate beyond three centimeters, and this forced the need for another C-section.

This was my wife, to whom I was married for 41 years, and who later died of a primary brain cancer at the age of sixty-two. Her brain cancer had no connection with her pregnancies. But this personal experience made me realize that a very healthy woman having a normal pregnancy can still have the risk of serious illness or death, even when there is excellent health care available.

Chapter 5: Medical Facts

At times, facts and statistics can be boring and make us fall asleep. Other times, we would prefer to not be bothered with the facts. But when we have important decisions to make, it is usually worthwhile to have as many facts as possible.

Whenever I was talking with one of my patients, I tried to explain the facts as clearly as possible. I always wanted to try to help my patients base their decision on what path was the most likely to have the best outcome for them. The only way to make that decision is to understand the risks and benefits of each option you have. Sometimes it made sense to take the riskier approach because of the benefit that might be derived. Other times, if you did not see any significant benefit, you certainly did not want to take any more risk than necessary. As with much of life, I saw different people interpret those risks and benefits differently based on their individual situation.

If you do not want to read the details and statistics, you can skip to the end of this chapter and read my summary.

When a woman becomes pregnant, whether planned or unplanned, she has a risk for both illness and death. Due to this, both state departments of health and the federal government, through the Centers for Disease Control and Prevention (CDC), have kept statistics on this issue:

- The CDC has a pregnancy mortality surveillance system (PMSS), which has been ongoing. The risk of death in the United States for a pregnant woman was 7.2 per 100,000 live births in 1987.
- By the year 2000, more than 14 women died for every 100,000 live births.
- In the year 2017, that figure was 17.3 women dying for every 100,000 live births.
- This is the number of women who die due to pregnancy either during or up to one year after birth if it is due to a pregnancy-related health issue. This ratio is called the PRMR (pregnancy-related mortality ratio).

Maternal mortality rates for pregnancy have been higher in the United States than in other developed countries. According to Roosa Tikkanen et al. (1), in 2018, there were 17 women who died for every 100,000 live births in the United States. This is very nearly the same as the 2017 rate, but this is twice or more compared to the rate in most other high-income countries. In contrast, this figure was three or less in the Netherlands, New Zealand, and Norway in the same year.

Even though we in the United States spend up to two times the cost for our health care, in some ways we do not have better health or even equal health compared to those other high-income countries.

A Woman Can Die from Pregnancy for Many Reasons

1. One example is the condition called *pre-eclampsia*, in which a woman develops hypertension, usually in the third trimester. If the condition is untreated, there is a higher chance it will become eclampsia, which can include seizures as well as death for the woman. With lack of prenatal care, there is a much greater chance it is not diagnosed and treated.

   NOTE: The lack of universal health insurance in our country contributes to a higher incidence of this type of problem. When a woman does not have health insurance, it is much more likely that she starts prenatal care late or presents to the hospital in labor without any prenatal care whatsoever.

2. *Ectopic pregnancy* occurs when implantation of the fertilized egg does not occur in the uterus

but occurs outside of the uterus, such as in the Fallopian tube or in the abdominal peritoneum. Because the growth of the placenta cannot occur as it normally does in the uterus, ectopic pregnancy nearly always results in the death of the embryo or fetus. It is also a high risk for the death of the mother, most often due to bleeding complications that can occur even before a woman knows she is pregnant. As a family physician, I had several patients who had ectopic pregnancies—and they could have easily died if they had not received quick diagnosis and management of their situations.

3. A third cause of death and disability in pregnant women is venous thromboembolism: blood clots in the legs and the lungs. Women are up to five times more likely to develop deep venous thrombosis (DVT) during pregnancy than when not pregnant (2). If a blood clot breaks off and travels to the lungs, this is called pulmonary embolism (PE). A large PE can stop oxygenation of the blood in the lungs and cause sudden death. The above article notes that PE is the leading cause of maternal death in the developed world. At the same time, hemorrhage (that is, bleeding) is the leading cause of maternal death in the developing nations.

Any doctor can tell you that diagnosing leg blood clots as well as blood clots in the lungs can be notoriously difficult. Ultrasound is commonly used in the United States to diagnose the leg blood clots. PE is usually diagnosed by contrast imaging using CAT (computerized axial tomography) scans, which are x-ray machines that use computerization to create multiple pictures to look at an area from multiple perspectives. Neither are readily available in developing countries.

Swelling in the leg is a common symptom of DVT. But leg swelling is common in the third trimester. As the fetus gets larger, there is more pressure on the veins that return blood to the heart and thus more chance that a woman's legs are swollen. That swelling is not always symmetrical. There are many times that it is not a simple decision as to whether to order an ultrasound for leg swelling in a woman in her third trimester of pregnancy.

4. A fourth example of how a woman can die from pregnancy is severe bleeding after delivery of an infant. The process of delivery of an infant can be going along entirely normally, and then uterine atony can occur. In uterine atony, the muscle of the uterus goes limp, and there is nothing to stop the vast flow of blood from the surface of the uterus. This happens more often with a large infant and difficult delivery but can also occur with an average-size infant. As soon as the infant is born, a woman is normally given either an

injection of oxytocin or an infusion of such medication through an intravenous line. Oxytocin is a hormone released by part of the brain in response to nipple stimulation, such as when a woman breastfeeds. But even when the injection or infusion occurs right after birth, severe uterine atony sometimes occurs.

As a resident doctor in family medicine, I was taught in such a situation to do manual massage of the uterus—you put one hand on the woman's abdomen and several fingers (gloved) in the vagina, then massaged the uterus to encourage it to contract. Most of the time those two measures stop the excessive bleeding. However, there are circumstances where an immediate consultation with an obstetrician is needed, and a hysterectomy can be required to save the life of the woman. This is an example of a potential complication that made me leery of the concept of home deliveries of infants. To be sure, it is not a frequent complication. But you cannot always predict who may be at higher risk.

It is remarkable how quickly a normal woman with normal blood clotting mechanisms can become hypotensive because of blood loss from either ectopic pregnancy or from uterine bleeding immediately after the birth of a child.

Pregnancy and childbirth are not without risk for a woman.

Roosa Tikkanen et al. (1) in their publication, *Maternal Mortality and Maternity Care in the United States Compared to 10 Other Developed Countries* point out:

- In the U.S., about one-third of pregnancy-related deaths occur during pregnancy
- 17 percent occur on the day of delivery
- 52 percent occur after birth
- 19 percent occur during the first week after birth, about one-fifth occur during the next five weeks
- 12 percent occur during the remainder of the year following childbirth
- The U.S. is the only high-income country that does not guarantee paid leave to mothers after childbirth
- Postpartum home visits are associated with improved mental health and breastfeeding outcomes, as well as reduced health care costs

The authors state, "All countries, apart from the U.S., guarantee at least one such visit within the first week postpartum."

They conclude, "While the reasons behind the high U.S. maternal mortality rate are multifaceted, our findings suggest that an undersupply of maternity providers, especially midwives, and lack of access to comprehensive postpartum supports are contributing factors."

In the practice I retired from in 2020, we had family physicians who delivered babies, as well as midwives, and both had access to immediate obstetrical consultation where an obstetrician was in the hospital 24 hours per day, 7 days per week, for those emergency cases to give the best outcome possible.

According to the CDC Pregnancy Mortality Surveillance System, there is significant difference in the PRMR (the risk of death from pregnancy) in different races or ethnicities in our country.

- The risk for non-Hispanic White women in 2014–2017 was 13.4 per 100,000 live births
- At the same time, the rate for Hispanic or Latino women was 11.6
- For non-Hispanic American Indian or Alaska natives, the rate was 28.3
- For non-Hispanic Black women, it was 41.7 per 100,000 live births

In other words, the risk of dying in our country if you are a pregnant Black woman is more than three times the risk of dying from pregnancy if you are a White woman. Likely many factors contribute to this difference, including 1) various access to health care, 2) different levels of health care insurance coverage, 3) behavioral patterns in both patients and in their care providers, and 4) social customs in different ethnic groups, as well as 5) the possibility of genetic factors affecting the risk of disease processes.

According to a study published in the journal *Obstetrics & Gynecology* in February of 2012, the risk of death for a woman in the United States from induced abortion is 0.6 per 100,000 abortions (3). The authors state that legal, induced abortion is markedly safer than childbirth. The risk of death associated with childbirth is approximately 14 times higher than with abortion. Similarly, the overall morbidity or illness associated with childbirth is greater than with abortion. Additional studies confirm that the risk of death from induced abortion in the U.S. is less than 1 per 100,000 abortions (4, 5), significantly safer than carrying a pregnancy to term.

If we wish to benchmark ourselves compared to other countries of the world, we can look at the statistics maintained by the World Health Organization (WHO). This organization uses the term *maternal mortality ratio* (MMR). It is defined as the ratio of maternal deaths per 100,000 live births. Maternal deaths are defined as deaths while a woman is pregnant or within 42 days of the end of pregnancy, irrespective of the duration and "site of pregnancy" from any cause related to or aggravated by the pregnancy, but not from accidental or incidental causes. The "site of pregnancy" is normally the uterus but can be the Fallopian tube or the abdominal peritoneum in the case of ectopic pregnancy, as earlier discussed.

According to the WHO:

- The MMR dropped 38 percent worldwide between 2000 and 2017.

- The MMR in low-income countries in 2017 was 462 per 100 000 live births versus 11 per 100,000 live births in high-income countries.
- So, the risk of death from pregnancy can be *20 to 40 times higher* in a low-income country versus high-income countries.
- But even in countries with the lowest MMR, the risk of death from pregnancy is not zero.

In a 2017 report by the WHO regarding maternal health, the MMR decreased from 7 in 2000 to 4 by 2017 in the European Union. The MMR for the Commonwealth of Independent States (CIS) had decreased from 36 to 16 during the same period.

According to a report published in the journal *Lancet Global Health* in September 2020 (6):

- Between 2015 and 2019, there was a yearly average of about 73 million induced (safe and unsafe) abortions worldwide.
- 39 induced abortions occurred per 1,000 women between 15 and 49 years of age worldwide. That is, about *one in 25 women* in this age group has an abortion within a year's time.
- This same report stated that almost one-third (29 percent) of all pregnancies, and *61 percent of all unintended pregnancies worldwide*, ended in induced abortion.
- So, the issue of abortion is a common one both in the United States and around the world.

Another report (7) estimated that between 2010 and 2014, about 45 percent of the induced abortions worldwide were *unsafe abortions*.

According to a fact sheet from the WHO dated September 25, 2020, abortions are safe when they are conducted by a person with the necessary skills, using a WHO-recommended method appropriate to the pregnancy duration. Also, almost every abortion death and disability could be prevented through sexuality education, use of effective contraception, provision of safe, legal induced abortion, and timely care for complications (8).

Abortion is not contraception. Contraception is for the prevention of pregnancy, but no method of contraception works all the time.

SUMMARY: Women can and do die from pregnancy. Induced abortion, when done by a trained healthcare professional using a medically appropriate method, especially in early pregnancy, is safer than carrying a pregnancy to term. This does not mean that every pregnant woman should consider abortion. It just means that in an unintended pregnancy, *it is appropriate for a woman to consider the risks and benefits of the options that she has.*

Case #2

A 28-year-old married Black woman is being followed for her first pregnancy and is about one month from her due date. Her pregnancy has been uncomplicated. She likes her family physician but has been reluctant to contact the clinic at times because she knows how busy her doctor is. She has an appointment today to start weekly checks in this last month before her due date. Just before she leaves to go to the clinic, she is called to reschedule her appointment for later in the week because her doctor just got called out of the clinic to go deliver another patient at the hospital. She has been having some swelling in the last week in both of her legs and understands that is normal. But she was going to ask today about one leg seeming to be more swollen than the other. The next evening, she starts having some chest pain when she breaths—and starts feeling a little anxious. She and her husband both think she should go to the emergency room for evaluation. After she gets there and is being evaluated, she has a sudden massive pulmonary embolus. The ER and obstetrical staff try to resuscitate her but are unsuccessful, and she and her infant both die. This case is a composite from cases that have been reported in medical journals.

Chapter 6: Genetic and Other Fetal Abnormalities

Certain genetic and developmental abnormalities are not usually compatible with ongoing life after birth. Trisomy 18 is such an anomaly. A different anomaly, trisomy 21, has more commonly been heard about—but there is far more variety in the severity of trisomy 21. Trisomy 21 is Down's syndrome, in which each cell has three number 21 chromosomes instead of the usual two. The wide range of situations in trisomy 21 is at least partly because mosaic trisomy 21 exists. This means some of the cells in the person's body do not have trisomy 21 and some cells do. The higher the percentage of normal cells, the less impact that trisomy 21 has on the individual's life. The individual with pure trisomy 21 usually has a number of severe issues—and the effect on neurologic development is the worst.

Trisomy 18 is a far more severe anomaly, which occurs in one in about 5,000 live births. A higher percentage of fetuses are affected, but some result in spontaneous abortion due to the developmental defects. When miscarriage (or spontaneous abortion) occurs early, a woman usually does not know that it was a genetic abnormality because there is often no evaluation of the tissue that is miscarried. With trisomy 18, many die before birth, or are stillborn, or die within the first month after birth. Many developmental defects are common in trisomy 18, such as heart defects, a small and abnormally shaped head, a small jaw and mouth, and clenched fists with overlapping fingers. In the 5 to 10 percent of individuals with trisomy 18 who live past one year of life, many have severe intellectual disability.

Does God cause an individual embryo or fetus to have trisomy 18? I cannot fathom a loving God would cause this to happen. But I do believe God is there to help the woman and her family deal with the tragic consequences of that chromosomal abnormality.

I cannot believe God would think it is wrong to terminate this pregnancy with the knowledge we have.

I understand some "pro-life" individuals believe God thinks it is wrong to terminate that pregnancy.

• Anencephaly is a serious birth defect in which a baby is born without parts of the brain and skull. According to a fact sheet from the CDC, it occurs in about 1 out of 4,600 births in the United States. It is a type of neural tube defect that can occur as the embryo develops. In the embryo, when the neural tube forms, if it does not close as usual, the fetal brain, spinal cord, and bones do not develop in the usual fashion. The cause of anencephaly in most infants is not known. Getting enough folic acid before and during early pregnancy can help prevent neural tube defects, such as anencephaly. Since the United States started fortifying grains with folic acid, there has been a 28 percent decline in pregnancies affected by neural tube defects, including spina bifida and anencephaly.

Anencephaly can be diagnosed during pregnancy or after the baby is born. During pregnancy, screening tests can be used to check for this birth defect and other conditions. Anencephaly could be suggested by an abnormal result on a blood or serum screening test, or it might be seen during an ultrasound (sounds waves are used to create pictures of the body). There is no known cure or standard treatment for anencephaly. Almost all babies born with anencephaly will die shortly after birth. Because a woman would still have the risks of pregnancy and the risk of death from childbirth, it is not unusual for a woman to have an abortion if she learns her fetus has anencephaly. This usually is not learned until the second trimester or later.

• Hydrocephalus is an abnormal buildup of cerebrospinal fluid in the ventricles of the brain that can occur as a developmental abnormality in the fetus. It can also occur for various reasons in children and adults. In the fetus, there is usually not an effective safe way to drain the fluid and remove pressure from the brain or treat whatever the underlying cause is. So, severe hydrocephaly can cause severe impairment of brain function. If the fetal head is larger than average due to this condition, this can also affect the risk of labor and delivery for the mother. So, the woman can have an increased risk of birth trauma at the same time the child would have a significant chance of being vegetative.

What if there is no rape, no incest, no chromosomal or developmental abnormality? Does God intend for every pregnancy to result in a healthy baby and healthy mother? If so, then why do chromosomal abnormalities such as trisomy 18 occur? Why do some mothers die from causes such as ectopic pregnancy? And why would this occur to a mother who already has children who need her to take care of them?

Certainly, the world is not ideal. It is not perfect. I do not accept the belief that God is choosing to cause harm to those beings that God has created. The loving God I know would not purposely cause such disaster for those He created and loved. But I do believe God is there to help us deal with these tragedies in life when or if they occur.

Case #3

Kathy, a 40-year-old married woman, is several months overdue for her menstrual period. She already has three children by a previous marriage and was not planning to get pregnant. She and her current husband used condoms most of the time. She has had some irregular periods, so at first, she was not thinking she could be pregnant, but then her pregnancy test is positive. She is worried about the increased risk of Down's syndrome. She is already very busy with the three children that she has. She does not think she would be able to care for an infant with that condition. But she also does not think she can undergo an abortion. She has been raised Catholic—and knows her church teaches that abortion is wrong. Genetic amniocentesis is a procedure in which a needle is introduced through a woman's abdominal skin, through the wall of the uterus, and into the fluid surrounding the fetus to obtain a sample of that fluid, which can then be tested to determine if the fetus has a genetic abnormality such as Down's syndrome. Genetic amniocentesis has a small risk (about 1–3 out of 1,000) of causing miscarriage.

The risk of having an infant with Down's syndrome for a woman at age 40 is about 1 in 85. If she were age 45, the risk would be about 1 in 35. After receiving counseling regarding all her options, she decides to not have genetic amniocentesis—and hopes her child will be normal.

What do you think you would have done?

When she gives birth, she has a healthy female infant. This case was an actual patient of mine and occurred over 30 years ago. The name was changed to protect the individual's privacy.

Chapter 7: Methods of Contraception

According to Contraceptive Technology (9), there are three general tiers of the various methods of contraception. In the third tier, and the least reliable, are the male and female condoms, diaphragms, withdrawal, the sponge, spermicides, and fertility awareness methods. The theoretical effectiveness of a method of birth control is often better than the real-world effectiveness. In general, the methods in the third tier have 13 or more pregnancies occur per 100 women per year.

In the second tier, which includes the ring, the patch, the pill, and injectables, about 4–7 unintended pregnancies occur per 100 women per year.

In the first tier, which includes implants, IUDs (intrauterine devices), vasectomies, or tubal ligation, less than one pregnancy happens per 100 women per year.

The key concept is that *all methods of contraception have some level of failure*, and thus unintended pregnancy occurs. All methods of contraception also have some risk of side effects. While it is safer to use contraception than to become pregnant, it is not risk free. Since there is not any 100 percent effective or risk-free method of contraception, the question becomes, "What options does a woman have—or should she have—when unintended pregnancy occurs?"

• Withdrawal is the method in which the man withdraws his penis from the woman's vagina prior to ejaculation. There are several reasons why this is an unreliable method. First, sperm may be present in the initial seminal fluid prior to ejaculation. Secondly, at the time of ejaculation, the strong emotions for both the male and female may prevent withdrawal from occurring even when it was strongly intended.

• Fertility awareness methods, including the rhythm method, are based on the concept of ovulation occurring for the woman at about day 14 of the ideal 28-day cycle. There is a slight change in the woman's basal body temperature at the time. There is a surge of luteinizing hormone (LH), which induces ovulation. Some women are very regular in their cycle, which helps when one is using this method. But because all women can have an irregular cycle and can have ovulation occur outside an ideal cycle, it is simply not as reliable as other methods. Also, many women have a stronger urge to have intercourse at mid-cycle due to the effects of LH on brain and body function.

• The male condom is used by many couples. In addition to a measure of protection against pregnancy, barrier methods of contraception do also reduce the risk of some sexually transmitted diseases. But the condom can break, can slip off, and can be forgotten when your mind is thinking about other issues.

• The diaphragm is a barrier device usually combined with a spermicidal jelly that is inserted in the woman's vagina and fits over the cervix. For many, it takes some practice to be able to place and remove the diaphragm. It requires a clinician visit because the appropriate size of the diaphragm is different for different women. Instruction on usage occurs with the visit for fitting the diaphragm. Although not common, the diaphragm can break like the condom can. It also must be used every time intercourse occurs.

• The birth control pill has been one of the most widely used methods of contraception since its initial approval by the FDA in 1960 (10). There are two main types of pills. The combined estrogen-progesterone pill is most commonly used. It is slightly more effective than the progesterone-only pill. A woman usually still gets her menstrual flow or period, but it is often less flow. For women with a heavy period, this can be a helpful feature. The estrogen component is responsible for certain possible side effects, such as the risk of venous thromboembolism (clot) or pulmonary emboli. It can increase the risk of migraine headache for some women. Some women can develop hypertension from the pill. The progesterone-only pill does not usually trigger migraine headaches. However, there is the chance of irregular bleeding on this type of pill. Overall, for most women, it is safer to use the birth control pill than it is to get pregnant. Injectable progesterone, such as Depo-Provera, is an intramuscular injection given about every three months at a clinic. If a woman is late to get the injection, the effectiveness decreases.

• Intrauterine devices (IUDs) have been available for many years, but the complications associated with one type—the Dalkon shield—reduced the popularity for a long time. The Dalkon shield was associated with a higher risk of pelvic inflammatory disease (PID). Newer IUDs have not been associated with PID but require a clinic visit for placement and for removal by a clinician. Due to the high level of effectiveness, and the fact they can last for 3–10 years depending on the type, they are the method of choice for some women.

• Implants of hormonal substances such as levo-norgestrel or etonogestrel are also highly effective. They are usually inserted subcutaneously in the skin of the forearm, which can be done as a procedure in a clinic. Implanon is a brand approved by the FDA in 2006, and it continues to be in use today in the United States. It is removed three years after placement but can be replaced if the patient desires to continue the same method.

• Vasectomy is the procedure in which a man's vas deferens are tied off to keep the sperm from flowing from the testes downstream. It is intended to be a permanent procedure but can fail, though it rarely does. Before relying on this method, one needs to have semen analysis done several months after the procedure to verify that sterility has been achieved.

I performed about one thousand vasectomies over the course of my years in practice. I always emphasized the need to have the semen analysis done to verify that the system had been cleared out. It was interesting how, despite that emphasis, some men never had the follow-up semen analysis.

I had a longtime patient (who did not have a vasectomy) who was an ardent "pro-life" individual. He had a cardiac valve problem and had to have heart surgery to replace the valve. Even though I did not do his surgery, he would often come in and tell me I saved his life because I had made the diagnosis and referred him to a cardiac surgeon. However, at some point, he learned I did vasectomies—which he thought was terrible. He was a Catholic and believed it was against God's will to use contraception of any type. He wrote me a letter to strongly encourage me to discontinue doing vasectomies. While I respected his individual belief, I did not stop doing vasectomies.

• Tubal ligation is the equivalent procedure in the woman, intended to prevent the eggs from traveling from the ovaries to the uterus. It requires an outpatient surgical procedure. When a couple is sure they do not want to have more children, either vasectomy or tubal ligation is commonly done. My wife Jane had a tubal ligation at the same time as her third C-section. If a woman needs multiple C-sections and is sure she has had all the children she wants, it is common to do a tubal ligation at the same time as her last C-section. I would have had a vasectomy if she had not been having that third C-section.

This is not meant to be an exhaustive list of all the methods of contraception or all the risks and benefits of each method. The main point is that all methods of contraception have their pros and cons. No method is perfect. Every method has a chance of some type of side effect or failure. When contraception fails, the result is unintended pregnancy. As earlier discussed, when unintended pregnancy occurs, the options are 1) to keep the pregnancy and resultant child, 2) to keep the pregnancy and give the child up for adoption, or 3) to have an abortion.

The raw statistics show that it is safer for the average woman to have an abortion than to carry a pregnancy to term, whether that pregnancy is intended or unintended. Certainly, this does not mean everyone should consider abortion. But when various laws are discussed that claim to promote women's health, this fact does not seem to be considered very often.

Case #4

Jasmine, a 19-year-old woman, has used oral contraception for several years, as it helps with her painful periods, called *dysmenorrhea.* She is attending college and enjoying both developing her relationship with her boyfriend as well as her studies.

Although she is usually very faithful in taking her pill, she forgets one day. She doubles up the next day when she realizes she forgot. She does not get her period when she expects to get it, but this has happened a few times since she has been on the pill. In the past, she would know she could not be pregnant, but since she and her boyfriend had started having intercourse, she was concerned. She goes to the student health clinic, and the result of her pregnancy test is positive. She feels she can discuss this with her boyfriend as well as her family (in many cases, this might not be reality). She knows she is not ready to be a mother. While she appreciates her boyfriend's support, she thinks he is also not ready to be a father. She knows that while most pregnancies result in a healthy mom and healthy baby, she does not want to take on the increased risks that occur in pregnancy. Her faith and religion teach her that life is to be respected—both her life and the life of the developing fetus. Her faith and religion teach her she has the option to decide what she thinks is best to do. She chooses to have a medical abortion at a clinic providing this service.

What do you think you would have done?

Chapter 8: Methods of Induced Abortion

Medical as well as surgical techniques are used for induced abortion.

The article "Modern Methods to Induce Abortion: Safety, Efficacy and Choice" contains a thorough review of the subject (11). Please refer to that article for any more details on any of these subjects in this chapter.

The use of medication has become much more common in the last 15 years. This method can be done at any stage of pregnancy, according to the WHO publication "Safe abortion: technical and policy guidance for health systems (2012)." The most effective regimen utilizes a combination of mifepristone, a progesterone receptor antagonist, followed by misoprostol, a synthetic prostaglandin E1 analog (12).

A systematic review of the method of using 200 milligrams oral mifepristone, followed by 800 micrograms of misoprostol administered buccally (held between the cheek and teeth) 24–48 hours later, in pregnancies up to

63 days gestation, documented an effectiveness of 96.7 percent among 33,846 women (13).

Prior to the availability of medical methods, uterine aspiration or suction by manual or electric vacuum has been used for pregnancies up to about 14 weeks gestation. Dilation and evacuation (D & E) is used from 14 to about 24 weeks gestation. Both methods are used when there is failure of the medical method—which is infrequent. Both methods are usually outpatient procedures in which the patient goes home the same day the procedure is performed.

In the case of uterine aspiration or suction, a paracervical block can be administered with local lidocaine-type anesthesia. The medication is injected in several locations at the edge of the cervix, which is the lowest part of the uterus and is visible from the vagina on pelvic examination. Sedation can be used if desired or needed by the patient but is not necessary. A good paracervical block prevents any sensation in most women for this procedure. If needed, the cervix is dilated, and then a fixed or flexible cannula or tube is passed through the cervical opening. Manual and electric suction each have their pros and cons. Manual suction may be quieter, depending on the motor used for electric suction.

Uterine aspiration or suction is safer and less painful than the older technique of dilation and sharp curettage or scraping (D & C) and is therefore the most widely recommended and utilized method of inducing abortion surgically in the first trimester (8).

In general, when an abortion is done at an earlier gestational age, the risk is less. In late pregnancy, the risk of abortion approximates the risk of childbirth.

Case #5

A 25-year-old unmarried woman has an appointment to determine whether she is pregnant. She has not had her menstrual period and had stopped taking the birth control pills prescribed at her well exam earlier in the year. She talks about her situation nonchalantly and does not show any emotion. From a past visit, I understand that she was abused physically as a child. Her pregnancy test is positive. Her uterine size on the pelvic exam is consistent with about a 12-week pregnancy. She does not have any ongoing relationship with the man who likely caused the pregnancy—and does not feel like she needs to consider his thoughts. She wants to discuss her options.

We review the possibilities of keeping the pregnancy and the infant, giving the infant up for adoption, or pursuing an abortion. This was in the 1980s when there was no medical option for abortion, only the surgical option. I did not encourage or discourage my patients from pursuing abortion or keeping the pregnancy. I tried to understand what the woman believed—and to understand her situation and explain the risks and benefits of each of the alternatives as best I could in the context of her situation. She was unsure what she wanted to do and left the office saying she would let me know. I learned later she pursued an abortion at a clinic in the metropolitan area.

What do you think you would have done?

Chapter 9: The "Pro-Life" Position

Those who believe that induced abortion is ethically wrong, and should be illegal, are commonly referred to as being "pro-life." Some pro-lifers believe an exception should be made in the cases of rape, incest, or severe genetic abnormalities. Some pro-lifers do not believe any exceptions should be made. Whether in the traditional Roman Catholic faith, or in some Protestant denominations, some believe God is against all induced abortions. Some believe God specifically creates each fertilized egg that has the chance to become a human being. Commonly, pro-lifers will state or believe "life" begins at the moment of conception. A "pro-choice" person would say in the vast majority of situations that a "pro-life" person is anti-abortion.

If I believed as these "pro-life" individuals believe, then I might be as passionate as some of them are in terms of trying to prevent any abortions. But I do not believe *making abortion illegal or putting restrictions on access to abortion is the best way to reduce the number of abortions.* If all people have contraception available and are educated in the usage of whatever method they use, that alone will reduce the number of unintended pregnancies. By doing so, there would be fewer pregnancies with genetic or developmental abnormalities, but it will certainly not eliminate the issue for the unfortunate women who have that occur.

I have often thought the best foreign policy investment our country could make would be to offer to pay for contraception in those countries which do not have the financial resources to do that for their citizens. Obviously, no contraception should be forced or mandated. Reducing the rate of unintended pregnancy worldwide—and being willing to give to poorer countries in this fashion—would be a useful and practical bit of foreign policy. I think we would get more bang for our buck than we get with many foreign policy initiatives.

While I respect that some people believe "life" starts at the moment of conception, I must explain why I do not believe this. I certainly believe God created this world, including the amazing DNA/RNA code that governs all life and all species. Without this chemical code, there would not be a mechanism for the transfer of all the methods by which life persists in so many different environments on planet Earth. Through the amazing gain in knowledge in genetics during my lifetime, we know each human being has a unique genetic code. Even identical twins can have minor differences in their genetic code. This is due to changes in the genetic code occurring after fertilization of the egg, and after the split of that early tissue into two individuals, causing identical twins. All of us have changes in the genetic structure of some of our cells as we age, since the reproduction of the DNA occurring during cell replication is not always a perfect process.

Before and after the moment of conception—fertilization of the egg with a sperm—there is life in both the egg and in the sperm. The question is whether this fertilized egg is a person in the same sense you and I are a person. The question is whether this biological entity warrants the same legal rights you and I have as a person. Given that the fertilized egg requires implantation in the uterus plus a gestation period of about nine months, the other question is whether this fertilized egg and potential subsequent embryo and fetus should have the same legal rights when its existence is totally dependent on the woman and the uterus in which it exists.

Ideally, every pregnancy would be planned, desired, and involve a normal fetus—but that is not reality.

When I think of a person, I think of their soul. I believe a person's soul exists before and beyond the existence of the physical human body. As a Christian, I believe when I die, my soul continues to exist, and God has said there is a place in heaven for each one of us.

Ask yourself:

- ✓ Does the soul enter the body at the moment of fertilization of the egg by the sperm?
- ✓ Does the soul enter at some point during the pregnancy?
- ✓ Does the soul enter at the moment of birth?

If the soul enters the body at the moment of fertilization or sometime during pregnancy, and if a woman has an abortion, I cannot believe a loving God would not take care of a soul that was God's creation.

I understand the "pro-life" person would say that an abortion results in the death of the fetus every time. When safe abortions are not available to the women who wish to have one, more unsafe abortions happen, and more women die as a result. For those women who already have children, more children lose their mother to death. And remember from the chapter on facts, more women die from pregnancy and childbirth than die from safe induced abortions.

When a woman wants to become pregnant and wants to have a child, a woman accepts the risk of pregnancy and childbirth. However, when a woman does not want to become pregnant, but has been raped and is pregnant due to this traumatic and illegal event, does society have the right to tell the woman that she must bear this excess risk, carry a pregnancy to term, and go through childbirth? When the woman is a victim of incest, must she bear this excess risk?

Ask yourself: Does society have the right to force the woman to bear this excess risk even if her pregnancy is not the result of rape or incest?

I would ask the "pro-life" person whether they believe in freedom of religion in our country. Or do they believe our country should have a state-sanctioned religion that believes the life created at the moment of conception is a person with legal rights that supersede the rights of the woman who has the pregnancy in her body?

Case #6

One day when I was on call for my clinic, I was alerted that the paramedics were taking a 16-year-old girl to the hospital after she had delivered an infant at home by herself. Her parents did not even know she was pregnant. She had not received any prenatal care. It is unknown when she became aware she was pregnant. She had managed to hide this from her parents and from her school. After going through labor and delivery on her own in her bedroom at home, she walked downstairs with the infant in her arms. She was bleeding vaginally, and the placenta had not yet been delivered. Her parents called the paramedics, who took her to the hospital. I met them at the hospital to deliver the placenta and examine her for any sign of tearing from the delivery or other issues.

I understand she placed her infant up for adoption. I never saw her again. I do not know with certainty, but I think it is likely that she had much fear and anxiety in dealing with her unintended pregnancy. For whatever reason, she did not feel comfortable talking with either her parents or a healthcare professional whenever it was that she became aware of her pregnancy. This made me wonder if she had been a victim of rape or incest.

What do you think you would have done if you had been in her position?

Chapter 10: The "Pro-Choice" Position

Here is my effort at making the differences clear:

- The person who is "pro-choice" believes a woman should be able to decide whether to continue her pregnancy.
- The "pro-life" person would often say a person who is "pro-choice" is pro-abortion.
- Supporting the right of a woman to choose whether to keep a pregnancy does not mean you agree with all abortions.
- The "pro-choice" person does not believe society has the right to force a woman to carry a pregnancy to term when she does not wish to do so. This does not mean every woman with an unplanned pregnancy should get an abortion. It does mean each woman should be able to consult her physician and anyone she considers to be an appropriate counselor, who could be a family member or close friend.

- After such consultation, the "pro-choice" individual believes the decision whether to keep the pregnancy is solely for the woman to decide because it is her body which must manage the pregnancy.
- Currently, there is no viable method to transfer a pregnancy from one woman to another. While in vitro fertilization is a wonderful option for couples with certain types of infertility, there is no technology that can remove the implanted embryo or fetus from one woman's uterus and transplant that embryo of fetus to another woman's uterus. Even if that technology existed, it would mean some level of risk for the woman who was pregnant. The "pro-choice" person does not tell the "pro-life" person that they must consider abortion for themselves. But the "pro-life" person is basically telling the "pro-choice" person that they are wrong—and it should be illegal for them to consider something the "pro-choice" person considers to be their right.
- The "pro-life" movement likes to say the fetus is not a choice but is a human life. I respect that as their belief. They have every right to believe that for themselves.
  - Do they have the right to force all humans to believe the same way they do?
  - Do they have the right to take away freedom of religion from those who believe differently about the status of the fetus?

The most extreme "pro-life" position would outlaw abortion in all cases, no matter whether incest, or rape, severe fetal abnormalities—or the life of the mother were involved. The most extreme "pro-choice" position would allow a woman to consider abortion at any stage of pregnancy, no matter the situation.

Most people have a belief that is somewhere between those two positions. Most people never have to deal with the situations that cause some women and some couples to consider an abortion in the late second or third trimester of their pregnancy.

The "pro-choice" person may support a group such as Planned Parenthood, whose predecessor was founded in 1916. According to its current website, "Planned Parenthood believes that all people—of every race, religion, gender identity, ability, immigration status, and geography—are full human beings with the right to determine their own future and decide, without coercion or judgement, whether and when to have children." Because Planned Parenthood affiliates are one of the largest abortion providers in the United States, many "pro-life" activists believe Planned Parenthood is evil—and thus frequent demonstrations occur outside Planned Parenthood clinics.

I believe the moderate pro-choice position is more pro-life than the "pro-life" position is. I call this pro-choice/pro-life. I will explain further what this position supports in Chapter 16.

I ask the "pro-choice" person to try to understand the emotional turmoil a "pro-life" person feels when they consider the number of elective abortions occurring in our country and around the world. For that person, in their religious belief, a lot of "humans with potential" are dying prematurely due to abortion.

Case #7

A 30-year-old married woman has a planned pregnancy and has no high-risk factors. According to the American College of Obstetricians and Gynecology (ACOG), she should have at least one standard ultrasound during pregnancy, which is usually done between 18–22 weeks of pregnancy. A first-trimester ultrasound can be done, but it is not standard because it is too early to see many of the fetus's limbs and organs in detail. Her ultrasound is done at 18 weeks and shows an apparent cardiac abnormality—a ventricular septal defect—and the size of the fetus's head is smaller than expected for her gestational age, i.e., microcephaly. An amniocentesis is recommended, and when the results come back, it shows the fetus has trisomy 18, Edward's syndrome.

As discussed earlier, this syndrome is not rare.

- It is the second most common trisomy (after trisomy 21, which is Down's syndrome).
- About one in 5,000 babies are born with trisomy 18, according to WebMD. It occurs more commonly than that, but many times the fetus does not survive the second or third trimester.
- According to WebMD, about half of babies with trisomy 18 who are carried full term are stillborn.
- The birthing process is still a risk for illness, injury, or death for the woman going through it.
- There is no cure for trisomy 18.

- The mother and father are counseled regarding the reality of trisomy 18. Her physician discusses the option of carrying the pregnancy to full term as well as the option of abortion. After further consideration of the options with their family as well as the pastor at their church, they decide to pursue abortion. Because this is late in the second trimester, the abortion must be done as a dilation and evacuation (D & E).

When the couple went to the clinic to have the abortion, protesters were outside the abortion clinic. One of them shouted, "Don't murder your baby!"

What do you think you would have done?

Do you think you have the option of telling this woman she cannot have an abortion?

Chapter 11: Roe v. Wade

The United States Supreme Court ruled on the case of *Roe v. Wade* on January 22, 1973. The case began in 1970 when "Jane Roe"—a fictional name used to protect the identity of the plaintiff, Norma McCorvey—instituted a federal lawsuit against Henry Wade, the district attorney of Dallas County, Texas, where Roe resided. The Supreme Court ruled 7–2 that unduly restrictive state regulation of abortion is unconstitutional.

In a majority opinion written by Justice Harry A. Blackmun, the court held that a set of Texas statutes criminalizing abortion in most instances violated a woman's constitutional right of privacy, which was found to be implied in the liberty guarantee of the due-process clause of the Fourteenth Amendment. The Fourteenth Amendment states, "Nor shall any state deprive any person of life, liberty, or property, without due process of law." (14)

The ruling considered three different stages of pregnancy and the resultant difference in the handling of the abortion issue with respect to constitutional and common law.

1. "For the stage prior to approximately the end of the first trimester, the abortion decision and its effectuation must be left to the medical judgment of the pregnant woman's attending physician."
2. "For the stage subsequent to approximately the end of the first trimester, the State, in promoting its interest in the health of the mother, may, if it chooses, regulate the abortion procedure in ways that are reasonably related to maternal health."
3. "For the stage subsequent to viability the State, in promoting its interest in the potentiality of human life, may, if it chooses, regulate, and even proscribe, abortion except where necessary, in appropriate medical judgment, for the preservation of the life or health of the mother."

Given the way the anti-abortion laws are written, **the issue is usually not the health of the mother—but the life of the embryo or fetus that is being considered**. Given the statistics regarding the risks of abortion versus childbirth I explained earlier, for most of pregnancy, it is safer for the woman to have an abortion than to carry the pregnancy to term.

I cannot think of another medical issue where the state takes away the right of the patient to decide what medical care to receive when various options are available. Even when lifesaving treatment is available, the state does not force an adult individual to get such treatment.

Controversy exists if the individual is a child—and the parents do not want the child to get the lifesaving treatment. If a child has insulin-dependent diabetes mellitus in which the administration of insulin is lifesaving, and if the child has parents who do not believe in the use of insulin for religious reasons, different legal cases have various outcomes. However, all would agree the child is a separate person, capable of living outside of the mother or father, but certainly requiring different levels of financial and social support, depending on the child's age and situation. Children have died due to the lack of use of insulin when their parents thought that praying to God or adequate faith would treat insulin-dependent diabetes mellitus. I think these results make it quite clear that God intends for us to use our brains and our medical knowledge.

In the abortion setting, the key issue is whether society, through the process of law, designates the embryo or fetus to be a legal person. Not only that, but the issue is whether the rights of the embryo or fetus—if it were designated as a legal person—can trump the rights of the woman in whose body the embryo or fetus must live.

In the situation where a woman believes the embryo or fetus is a person whose rights trump her own rights; it certainly makes sense that the woman should not or would not pursue an abortion. But does society have the right to tell all women that all embryos and fetuses have rights that trump the rights of pregnant women? This becomes an issue very much affected by religious beliefs.

Thus, the issue of freedom of religion is quite pertinent to the abortion issue in a legal sense. In reading the case of *Roe v. Wade*, I did not see any discussion regarding the issue of freedom of religion.

In the 1973 decision, Justice Blackman referred to the history of the position of the American Medical Association (AMA) regarding abortion. "The anti-abortion mood prevalent in this country in the late 19th century was shared by the medical profession. Indeed, the attitude of the profession may have played a significant role in the enactment of stringent criminal abortion legislation during that period." (14)

He further noted, "In 1970, after the introduction of a variety of proposed resolutions, and of a report from its Board of Trustees, a reference committee noted 'polarization of the medical profession on this controversial issue'; division among those who had testified; a difference of opinion among AMA councils and committees; 'the remarkable shift in testimony' in six months, felt to be influenced 'by the rapid changes in state laws and by the judicial decisions which tend to make abortion more freely available'; and a feeling 'this trend will continue.'" On June 25, 1970, the House of Delegates adopted preambles and most of the resolutions proposed by the reference committee. The preambles emphasized "the best interests of the patient," "sound clinical judgment," and "informed patient consent," in contrast to "mere acquiescence to the patient's demand."

The resolutions asserted that abortion is a medical procedure that should be performed by a licensed physician in an accredited hospital only after consultation with two other physicians and in conformity with state law, and that no party to the procedure should be required to violate personally held moral principles. (Proceedings of the AMA House of Delegates 220 – June 1970).

Given the statistics I quoted earlier regarding the safety of abortion from the 2012 study (3), and the fact that nearly all abortions are now done on an outpatient basis, it simply shows how the status of medicine has changed substantially since the early 1970s.

Then, it was thought it was necessary to do many medical procedures in the hospital—which are now routinely done on an outpatient basis due to progress in many areas of medicine.

In the early 1980s, it was routine to do cataract surgeries on the eyes as an inpatient, and the patient had to lie in bed for several days. Now, cataract surgery is nearly always done on an outpatient basis, and the person is routinely seen the following day in the office for a postoperative checkup. Sometimes even knee replacement surgeries are done on an outpatient basis. When hospitalization is needed after a knee replacement, it is common for a patient to be in the hospital for only one day after the procedure.

So it is with abortion—it is done safely as an outpatient procedure in most situations.

Today, per the AMA website, according to the Code of Medical Ethics Opinion 4.2.7, The Principles of Medical Ethics of the AMA do not prohibit a physician from performing an abortion in accordance with good medical practice and under circumstances that do not violate the law.

Just as in society as a whole, there have been and remain differences in opinion regarding abortion in the medical profession. One can debate the ethics of abortion or one's religious beliefs about abortion, but the medical facts regarding current abortion methods are straightforward.

Chapter 12: Religious Beliefs

As a family physician, I saw many pregnancies. When a woman wanted to be pregnant and was healthy and her fetus was healthy, it could be like a vision of heaven. When a woman had an unintended pregnancy or some illness or fetal abnormality, it could be like a vision of hell.

I will describe the beliefs of a few religions as best I understand them regarding abortion. As I said earlier, we cannot fully understand someone's situation unless we have been in the exact same situation.

The Roman Catholic Church

The formal teaching of the Roman Catholic Church is that God is against abortion, and it should not be performed. Various Protestant denominations of the Christian faith also believe this. At the same time, many Christian denominations believe it is appropriate for the woman to be able to choose whether to have an abortion in her situation. The views of other faiths, such as Judaism, Buddhism, Hinduism, or agnosticism, also matter in a country that states in the First Amendment to the Constitution that "Congress shall make no law respecting an establishment of religion or prohibiting the free exercise thereof."

The following is the position of the Roman Catholic Church as I understand it from various sources:

- The Roman Catholic Church says that deliberately causing an abortion is very wrong.
- The church bases this doctrine on natural law and on the written word of God.
- The Roman Catholic Church says human life begins when the egg is fertilized by male sperm.
- From the moment of conception, the Roman Catholic Church believes that a unique life begins, independent of the life of the mother and father.
- Each new life that begins at this point is not a potential human being but a human being with potential, according to the church.
- Since the sixteenth century, causing or having an abortion led to automatic excommunication.
- This is stated in the Code of Canon Law (1983): "A person who actually procures an abortion incurs automatic excommunication" (Canon 1398).

- The strong stance taken by the Roman Catholic Church has underpinned many of the pro-life groups that have been formed to challenge the legalization of abortion.

At the same time, many Roman Catholics believe that abortion should be legal in a variety of circumstances in our country. I have known many Roman Catholics on both sides of the aisle when it comes to this question.

In the previous description of the Roman Catholic Church position, the statement is made: From the moment of conception, the Roman Catholic Church believes that a unique life begins, independent of the life of the mother and father.

That is a key concept to me, because the life of the embryo or fetus is definitely not independent of the life of the mother. Until the time of birth, and even after birth, being pregnant is a definite risk to the life of the mother. If the woman has knowingly desired to get pregnant, it is an acceptable risk. When pregnancy was not intended, many times this pregnancy is not an acceptable risk.

I have been a member of the Evangelical Lutheran Church in America (ELCA) or its predecessor since I was born. As such, I am a Christian. The ELCA position on abortion was adopted at the 1991 ELCA Churchwide Assembly. The 12-page document explains there is much more to the issue than the brief "pro-choice" or "pro-life" labels. It states: "This church recognizes that there can be sound reasons for ending a pregnancy through induced abortion." It also states, "Induced abortion…is one of the issues about which members of the Evangelical Lutheran Church in America have serious differences." (15)

Jewish Point of View

In the July 24, 2019, issue of *USA Today,* an article was titled "Jews, outraged by restrictive abortion laws, are invoking the Hebrew Bible in the debate." (©Lindsay Schnell, USA Today Network) The article quotes Danya Ruttenberg, a Chicago-based rabbi who has written about Jews' interpretation of abortion. "It makes me apoplectic. Most of the proof texts that they're bringing in for this (to say that God is against abortion) are ridiculous. They're using my sacred text to justify taking away my rights in a way that is just so calculated and craven."

Across the country, as a wave of anti-abortion legislation reinvigorates the fight over reproductive rights, Jewish religious leaders, activists, and women are speaking out in favor of a woman's right to choose, buoyed by their faith.

It's not just that the U.S. shouldn't be deriving law from poetic language, Ruttenberg said. It's that the Jewish tradition has a distinctly different reading of the same texts. While conservative Christians use the Bible to argue that a fetus represents a human life, which makes abortion murder, Jews don't believe that fetuses have souls and, therefore, terminating a pregnancy is no crime.

Studies from the Pew Research Center show that Jews overwhelmingly (83 percent) support abortion rights. The National Council of Jewish Women, a 126-year-old organization that helped establish some of the first birth control clinics across the country, considers re-productive rights a cornerstone issue and has publicly condemned the strict abortion bans recently handed down in Alabama and Mississippi.

It's common in this debate to hear the Christian per-spective. But what's often left out of the conversation is how Jews, who read the Hebrew Bible—referred to in Christian circles as the Old Testament—argue that their tradition condones abortion. Sometimes, if the mother's life is at stake, it even insists on it.

"This is a big deal for us," Ruttenberg says. "We're very clear about a woman's right to choose. And we're very clear about the separation between church and state."

National Survey

The Pew Research Center, Washington, D.C., con-ducted a Religious Landscape Study in May of 2014. The survey questioned 35,000 Americans from all 50 states about their religious affiliations, beliefs, and prac-tices, as well as their social and political views. This in-cluded their views on abortion. The results regarding whether one believed most abortions should be legal, or illegal, were as follows:

Faith	Legal (%)	Illegal (%)	Don't Know (%)
Jewish	83	15	2
Buddhist	82	17	1
Unaffiliated	73	23	4
Hindu	68	29	3
Protestant	60	35	5
Muslim	55	37	9
Orthodox Christian	53	45	2
Historically Black Protestant	52	42	6
Catholic	48	47	5
Evangelical Protestant	33	63	4
Mormon	27	70	3
Jehovah's Witness	18	75	7

You can see in the above statistics that even in a faith such as the Catholic Church, there can be a difference between the formal church teaching by its leadership—and the thoughts of the members of the faith.

I have tried to understand where the "pro-lifer" finds the passages in the Bible that says to them that God thinks abortion is wrong. I do not find any passage speaking directly to the issue of potential induced abortion. At the time the various books of the Bible were written, elective induced abortion by a qualified physician did not exist.

Psalm 139 verse 13 is often referred to: "For you created my inmost being: you knit me together in my mother's womb" (The Life Application Bible: New International Version, published by Tyndale House Publishers, Wheaton, Illinois 1991). Since God is all-knowing, I presume God knows which pregnancies will result in spontaneous abortion. According to the "pro-life" belief, that is a person from the moment of conception through the time that spontaneous abortion or miscarriage occurs. If such a pregnancy is a person with a soul, I presume God takes care of this person. Is it possible that no fetus has a soul till either later in pregnancy or at the time of birth? Again, this returns to the issue of belief or faith in a given religion. There is not any scientific way to determine whether a fetus has a soul.

The Christian church has many different denominations. Some theologians will tell you God says abortion is wrong. Some theologians will tell you God does not say that abortion is wrong. Some say the Bible is the word of God recorded by man at God's direction. So, a variety of interpretations of the same document exist.

- Is one interpretation the correct one?
- Is one religion the correct one?

My father taught me that God is more than male or female—only God is God. The traditional Christian faith and church has been a patriarchy. Jesus's disciples were all male. The leadership of the Jewish church at the time of Jesus was male. All the leadership of the Roman Catholic Church is still male—there has been no female Pope, and all priests and bishops still must be male. Many Protestant denominations now allow male or female pastors and bishops. At the time of the founding of our country, in the initial United States Constitution, a woman's right to vote was not included. It took the approval of the 19th Amendment to the Constitution in 1920 to allow women to vote.

I wonder if women had written the Bible—how all this would have been handled.

I wonder what God thinks of all the different versions of the Bible that exist.

Chapter 13: Is Abortion Murder?

In some pro-life advertising, the statement is made that abortion is murder. Murder is commonly defined as the intentional unlawful killing of one person by another person. Stating that abortion is murder means you consider the fetus to be a person. A person is normally physically separate from another person. If one thinks abortion is murder, there is no consideration of the fact that the life of the fetus is totally dependent upon the woman's body—her uterus and supporting structures—for survival.

Some articles describing a biblical rational for the anti-abortion position state that the commandment, "You shall not murder," includes abortion. This assumes the individual separate human life begins at conception, and that the soul of an individual is also present at that point. As I have stated, many Christians, as well as members of the Jewish faith and other faiths, do not believe those assumptions.

If abortion is considered by some to be murder, then why not give contraception to all to reduce the risk of unintended pregnancy? But at least some of the "pro-life" group believe God decides when a woman becomes pregnant—and thus use of contraception would be against God's will. Again, the issue returns to the fact it is the religious belief of some people who believe their religious belief should trump the religious beliefs of the remainder of the population. To me, this clearly violates the United States Constitution's concept of freedom of religion. Thus, the answer to "Is abortion murder?" depends upon one's religious faith. Some will consider abortion to be murder while others will vehemently state that abortion is not murder—and that it is very wrong to use that term. If abortion is outlawed, then the religious faith that believes life begins at conception and is a legal person at the moment of conception becomes the state-supported religion. The separation of church and state that is supposed to exist in our country would no longer exist.

Case #8

A young family physician finished her three-year residency. During one rotation, she learned how to do abortions by the method of suction curettage. This is the same procedure used to stop bleeding for a woman with a spontaneous incomplete abortion that threatens her health and her life due to bleeding or infection. The physician knows it is worthwhile to be able to do the procedure for her patients who may need it. After she starts her medical practice with her new group, she has a patient with an unintended pregnancy—the woman is sure she wants to have an abortion. The physician counsels her patient on the risks and benefits of the options that exist. The young family physician is trained and qualified to do the procedure—and does it for the patient. Not long after that, she becomes aware of the threats made to some physicians who do abortions by "pro-life" supporters. She is married and has a young family. She does not want to have the chance that her family experiences violence or even her death as a result of a radical "pro-life" individual. She decides she will not do any further therapeutic abortions—and will refer her patients to an abortion clinic in the metropolitan area.

What do you think you would have done if you had been in the shoes of this young physician?

Dr. George Tiller, who was the only doctor who provided abortions at the time in Wichita, Kansas, was murdered on May 31, 2009, while ushering at a service at Reformation Lutheran Church in Wichita. He was shot in the head at close range, while wearing a so-called bullet-proof jacket. In 1998, after a doctor in New York state was killed by a gunman in his home, Tiller had been told by the FBI that he was No. 1 on the violent anti-abortionists' hit lists. (16)

An article in the *American Economic Journal* by Mireille Jacobson and Heather Royer (17), states: "Between 1973 and 2003, anti-abortion activists carried out over 300 attacks (arsons, bombings, and butyric acid attacks at abortion facilities, and the murder of abortion providers) on abortion clinics in the United States. The frequency of these attacks makes abortion clinic violence one of the most common forms of domestic terrorism in this country."

I find it difficult to understand how someone can say they are "pro-life," and then encourage and condone behavior such as the murder of a physician or the bombing of an abortion clinic. I understand many "pro-life" individuals do not accept or condone that behavior, but enough do accept it to cause the above. How many physicians and other health care workers have hesitated to either work at an abortion clinic or even talk about abortion due to the threat of violence? A group such as Operation Rescue, on its website, takes responsibility for closing abortion clinics and states it is doing the "Christian" thing, and quotes Bible verses to support its work. The God I know and love would not agree with the work of Operation Rescue.

So, does our country say that my form of Christianity is not okay?

Does our country have freedom of religion?

"Be kind and compassionate to one another, forgiving each other, just as in Christ God forgave you."
Ephesians 4:32 (NIV)

Chapter 14: Human Population and the Capacity of Planet Earth

If the "pro-life" or anti-abortion position were in effect around the world, more humans would be born in the short term. Facts today are:

- The earth's human population is projected to reach 8 billion people in 2023.
- It was only 1800 that the human population was around 1 billion. It took until 1927 for the population to double to 2 billion.
- By 1974, the population had doubled again to 4 billion.
- While the growth rate has declined over the last 30 years, the absolute increase in the human population continues to be substantial.
- The current average annual population growth is about 81 million people (18).

- In the period of 2015-2019, the annual number of abortions worldwide was estimated to be 73 million (6).

The size of the Earth is not growing, nor is the land surface available for producing food for human consumption. Many of our current significant world problems are at least partly due to overpopulation, straining the capacity of the world to support us.

Many immigrants came to the United States in the 1800s due to various famines and food shortages in European countries. Today, worldwide, we continue to see migration of the human population due to food scarcity in a variety of regions. As the population has increased, and the effect on the planet is more pronounced, we have only become more interdependent upon each other on planet Earth.

While it is hoped that we will find solutions to producing more food, dealing with global warming, reducing pollution, etc., all these problems are magnified by the issue of overpopulation. If we have more people die due to heat, pollution, famine, or diseases that are worsened due to crowding from overpopulation, then we are not loving our neighbor. For a Christian, according to Jesus, God's second commandment is to "Love thy neighbor as thyself."

If as a global society we keep our population voluntarily at a lower level, and we enable more people to live a long, healthy life, then over time, it is entirely possible that more humans inhabit the planet. If we do not voluntarily control our population, and the resultant overpopulation causes more premature death and misery, then it is possible that fewer humans ultimately inhabit the planet.

It is not my belief that God wants us to overpopulate the planet or destroy the world we have been given to live on. I believe God wants us to use the brains we have been given to solve all the above issues, and to enable us to have more humans live on planet Earth over a long time.

Again, *abortion is not a method of contraception*. It is an option for the woman who has an unintended pregnancy and decides she does not think it is best for her to carry her pregnancy to term. She alone can best decide what she should do. She certainly should consult her family and loved ones as she sees fit. But I do believe it is her body, and hence her decision to ultimately decide what is best to do. I do believe God gave each woman and each man a brain to be used to best decide how to manage a variety of situations.

Chapter 15: Insurance Coverage of Abortions and Contraception

If a woman with an unintended pregnancy believes that it is appropriate for her to pursue an abortion, she still must be able to get to a clinic that will perform the procedure—and then be able to pay for the procedure. For many women, their health insurance coverage through their employer covers such a reproductive health issue. But if a woman is poor, or does not have insurance, or works for a company whose insurance does not provide such a benefit, it may not be practical to consider this option. If a woman works for the federal government, is in the United States military, is in federal prison for whatever reason, or is a Peace Corps volunteer—her health insurance funded by the federal government does not contain coverage for abortion (19). In those circumstances, society is effectively telling the woman that abortion is not an acceptable option.

Medicaid is the federal program providing medical insurance for persons who are poor enough to qualify for it and do not have any other source of health insurance. There is federal funding of the program, although it is in conjunction with state law and state funding, so the criteria to qualify for Medicaid are different in all 50 states of the union. Following *Roe v. Wade* in 1973, abortions were covered by Medicaid. "Pro-life" individuals and organizations did not want their tax money paying for abortions. Similarly, individuals and organizations that are against war have not wanted their tax money to be spent on the military. But that group has not been successful in keeping the federal government from using their tax money for that purpose. The "pro-life" lobby has been very successful at keeping the federal government from spending federal tax money on abortions.

It is ironic that the Republican Party usually wants to keep the government out of the lives of private individuals. "Pro-life" individuals are a significant part of the supporters of the Republican Party. Through the policies and the laws that have been enacted due to this lobby, the government has a great deal of involvement in the personal decision-making of many women in our country.

After *Roe v. Wade* in early 1973, Medicaid paid for abortions for the women under this insurance. In 1976, the Hyde amendment was initially passed by Congress, which prohibited the use of federal funds to pay for any abortion under Medicaid (19). It was subsequently modified to allow for abortion if the pregnancy was the result of rape, incest, or if the life of the mother was in danger (19). Due to legal challenges, the Hyde amendment was not enforced until 1980, when the Supreme Court ruled that it was constitutional in the 5-4 decision *Harris vs. McRae* (20). From 1973, when abortion first became legal, until 1980, when the Hyde amendment first took effect, the joint federal-state Medicaid program was paying for roughly 300,000 abortions annually (19). The Hyde amendment is a rider to an annual appropriations bill, which means it is not permanent law and must be renewed each year.

Justice Brennan was one of the four dissenting justices in *Harris v. McRae*. In his dissent, he writes, "The Hyde Amendment's denial of public funds for medically necessary abortions plainly intrudes upon this constitutionally protected decision, for both by design and in effect it serves to coerce indigent pregnant women to bear children that they would otherwise elect not to have" (20).

Justice Marshal, another one of the four dissenting justices, adds, "Under the Hyde Amendment, federal funding is denied for abortions that are medically necessary and that are necessary to avert severe and permanent damage to the health of the mother. The court's opinion studiously avoids recognizing the undeniable fact that for women eligible for Medicaid—poor women—denial of a Medicaid-funded abortion is equivalent to denial of legal abortion altogether. By definition, these women do not have the money to pay for an abortion themselves. If abortion is medically necessary—and a funded abortion is unavailable, they must resort to back-alley butchers, attempt to induce an abortion themselves by crude and dangerous methods, or suffer the serious medical consequences of attempting to carry the fetus to term. Because legal abortion is not a realistic option for such women, the predictable result of the Hyde Amendment will be a significant increase in the number of poor women who will die or suffer significant health damage because of an inability to procure necessary medical services" (20).

By 1981, the only exception to the prohibition on abortion coverage under Medicaid that Congress allowed was for "the life of the mother" (19). This lasted until 1993, when Democrats had a majority in both the House and Senate, and President Clinton was an abortion-rights supporter. Rep. Hyde offered his amendment but changed the wording to include exceptions for rape and incest because "I didn't think the votes were there anymore for a straight ban on abortion funding." There were enough anti-abortion Democrats that his amendment with that wording was passed and has continued to be included in the annual appropriations bill (19).

The Affordable Care Act (ACA), formally known as the Patient Protection and Affordable Care Act, is also called Obamacare. It was enacted by the 111th Congress and signed into law by President Obama on March 23, 2010 (21). One feature of the act required employer-sponsored health care coverage to include coverage for all forms of contraception approved by the FDA. An exemption to contraception-coverage requirements was given to religious employers and non-profit religious institutions—but not to for-profit institutions. Various legal challenges have occurred to this mandate. In the case of Burwell vs. Hobby Lobby Stores, the Supreme Court in 2014 with a 5–4 vote ruled that "closely held, for-profit companies owned by individuals with religious objections did not have to directly provide contraceptive coverage to their employees" (22). "The Green family owns and operates Hobby Lobby Stores, Inc.…with over 500 stores and 13,000 employees. The Green family has organized the business around the principles of the Christian faith and has explicitly expressed the desire to run the company according to biblical precepts, one of which is the belief that the use of contraception is immoral" (23). While I respect the belief of the Green family and their desire to not cover contraception through the health insurance benefit of their closely held corporation, I must explain that this Christian faith is quite different from the Christian faith I am a part of. Most of the Christians I know believe it is perfectly appropriate to use contraception. Just as with the abortion issue, I am not able to find any verse in the Bible stating that God is against using contraception.

When I was forty years old, my mom gave me a study Bible called the Life Application Bible, New International Version (NIV). Over the course of about four years, I read the entire Bible and have reread numerous portions since then. I am not a Bible scholar, but certainly I saw no passages referring to contraception. Such technology did not exist two thousand years ago. However, numerous passages talked about how much God loves us. Also, numerous were other passages where God asks us to forgive others. In the Lord's prayer, there is the phrase "and forgive us our trespasses as we forgive those who trespass against us."

It does not make any sense that God would want us to not use contraception—then overpopulate the world and increase the probability of death and destruction for many people on our planet.

It is ironic that a policy such as that promoted by the above-mentioned family and its corporation would have the impact of increasing the number of abortions due to the higher incidence of unintended pregnancy when contraception is not used. I cannot believe that the God I know and love would agree with such a policy.

For many reasons, I think it is best for health insurance to be separated from employment. Perhaps it should be separated from government as well. From an actuarial and cost point of view, it is certainly cheaper to cover contraception and abortion than to not cover those. Pregnancy and labor, and delivery and health care of a child are certainly far more expensive than the alternative—which does not mean I am against having children. I love my children and grandchildren very much. It is simply that from a fiscal point of view, it makes sense to cover contraception and abortion for those individuals who feel those services are needed.

Case #9

A twenty-year-old woman has not had her period. Her periods are sometimes irregular, so at first, she was not concerned. Over a month ago, she went out to a bar with friends and woke the next morning not remembering the night before. She does not drink excessively and thinks someone slipped some type of medication into her drink. She was too ashamed to tell any of her friends about this. Her parents divorced when she was young, and she does not know her father. Her mother died from cervical cancer several years ago. She does a home pregnancy test—and it is positive. She works several part-time jobs and does not qualify for health insurance at any of her jobs and is still trying to pay off her debt at a hospital, where she had to have an emergency appendectomy a year ago. As far as she knows, she does not qualify for her state's Medicaid program, and even if she did, it does not cover abortions. She knows she is not ready to take care of a child and does not want to go through pregnancy. She heard through the grapevine that a person in an apartment building nearby could give her something that would cause an abortion. But she also heard one person who tried this got really sick and is no longer seen around the neighborhood. She also heard that hitting her lower abdomen could trigger an abortion. She does not know what to do.

What would you do if you were this person and in this situation?

Chapter 16: My Practical World

Every year worldwide, more than 60,000 women die from unsafe abortion (24). Whether in undeveloped countries or in developed countries, this is tragic. Studies have shown that abortion rates are similar in countries where abortion is highly restricted compared to where it is easily legally available (25). The main difference is that more abortions are unsafe in countries where abortion is very restricted. The more contraception and legal abortion are available, the lower the incidence of maternal mortality. In other words, *fewer women die when they have easy access to contraception as well as to legal abortion when unintended pregnancy occurs*.

I believe that pro-choice/pro-life is the path God wants me to pursue. This means I believe that all people should practice responsible sexual activity—in that contraception should be available and used when a couple is not trying to become pregnant. It is an appropriate function of government to ensure that all people have contraception available to them for this purpose. When a pregnancy is desired and pursued, then medically appropriate prenatal care should be followed by all women when pregnancy occurs, and their male partner should be supportive of all the healthy behaviors a woman needs to do to give the pregnancy the best chance of successful conclusion. This gives the best chance of a healthy baby being born to loving parents. There should be no coercion to have a pregnancy or the resulting baby for those who do not wish to have such. No law should encourage or discourage pregnancy and childbirth.

If every child were planned and desired, and society pursued all efforts to give each child the best chance of developing into a healthy adult, all of society would benefit. Because there would be far fewer unintended pregnancies, far fewer women would even need to consider abortion.

If an unintended pregnancy occurs—and a woman does not believe it is best for her to carry the pregnancy to term, I believe she has a right to have an abortion to terminate the pregnancy. I believe God loves her just as much as would be the case if she wanted to carry the pregnancy to term.

This should happen:
- She should be educated so she knows the signs of early pregnancy; then diagnosis occurs earlier, rather than later.

- She should be comfortable talking with her family and friends as needed as she decides what course is best for her to take.
- She should be supported by family, friends, and society in either course she takes.
- If her decision is for abortion, then I believe it is appropriate that society does not put any barriers in her path.
- If her decision is for continuing the pregnancy to childbirth, society should make sure that good prenatal care is available for her.
- If her decision is to keep the resulting baby and raise that child, then society should support her efforts on this path.
- If her decision is to give the child up for adoption, then society should support her decision and make the process as smooth as possible for both the woman and for the adoptive parents.

But every situation is not ideal. When a genetic abnormality such as trisomy 18 is diagnosed, it is commonly in the second trimester. If there are delays in diagnosis due to a variety of practical aspects, it can be diagnosed in the late second or early third trimester.

Various heart disorders, including abnormal heart valves, can significantly affect the risk of pregnancy for a woman. Severe mitral stenosis, which reduces blood flow between the left atrium and left ventricle of the heart, can be extremely risky and cause death for the pregnant woman, especially in the third trimester. Pregnancy is often not advised for a woman with this condition. It would help in this situation if contraception were always reliable—and had no side effects.

It is key that society should not interfere with the physician-patient relationship. The physician has a legal, moral, and ethical obligation to serve each patient in the best fashion possible. Medical knowledge changes, and laws cannot keep up with those changes. In our society, with freedom of religion, it is unacceptable and unreasonable for restrictions to be placed on medical practice—and on a woman's options—based on the religious beliefs of only a part of the population.

When a law is passed that claims to be concerned about a woman's health and the state's interest in protecting a woman's health—but in reality, increases the risk for a woman—this is clearly unconstitutional. Yet it has happened already with various restrictions on abortion existing in numerous states in our country. A woman with an unintended pregnancy—who has one of the above medical conditions and lives in a part of our country where there are significant restrictions on abortion care—has a higher risk of disability or death. This is at least part of the reason that the United States has more women die from pregnancy than other developed countries.

Because many different personalities and many different situations exist, there will always be the cases that test our beliefs in some fashion. What if a woman carries a pregnancy to the third trimester (last three months), and the woman and fetus are physically healthy—but then the woman wants to have an abortion? Because the fetus has a substantial chance of survival outside of the woman's uterus, I do not think the woman should be able to have an abortion so late in the pregnancy.

I understand a given woman may delay her decision for a variety of reasons. But I think once a pregnancy has reached the point of significant chance of viability outside the woman's body, then abortion should not be available. The exception would be the situation where a woman has a pregnancy with a high probability of fetal death or neonatal death such as trisomy 18 not diagnosed until the late second trimester or early third trimester. Another exception is the pregnancy in a woman who develops a medical condition that causes pregnancy to be a substantial risk to her life.

Chapter 17: Pro-Choice/Pro-Life

I believe that pro-choice/pro-life is the position that best describes what God desires for all of us to pursue.

This position gives human life the best chance at long-term success on planet Earth and thus best supports the sanctity of human life. I believe this position will result in the fewest abortions over the long haul because of an emphasis on appropriate contraception and a healthy attitude toward human sexuality. I believe God intended that we celebrate our sexuality as part of the amazing creation that we have been given. I believe God intends for us to be honest and straightforward, as well as respectful and loving in our sexual relationship.

This position advocates:

- For the availability of effective contraception for any man or woman who desires it.

- All persons have a responsibility to be honest and responsible in their sexuality in any relationship.

- Men have as much responsibility for contraception as women do.

- The appropriate use of contraception reduces the incidence of unintended pregnancy.

- When unintended pregnancy occurs, it is the responsibility of the person or persons affected to discuss with their health care provider and loved ones—and to decide the best course of action for the individual.

- When a woman affected by unintended pregnancy decides she does not believe it is best for her to carry her pregnancy to term, she has the right to pursue an abortion by the safest, most effective method of abortion available.

- Health care professionals have the right to provide such care to an individual who desires to pursue it.

- If a health care professional does not wish to participate in the delivery of care to such an individual, then at a minimum they have the responsibility to make that clear to the community they serve.

- In other words, someone who currently considers themselves to be "pro-life," such as a pharmacist, does not have the right to refuse to dispense a medication used for abortion—or they should tell their community what their belief is, and another pharmacist should always be easily available to a woman seeking to fill such a prescription.

If this is not what God wants me to do, then God has every right to judge me—but another human does not have the right to presume they have the correct interpretation of what God says is right. Another human is just as fallible as I am—even the Pope, for those who happen to be of the Catholic faith. No human is God—which is why we are supposed to have freedom of religion in our country.

Therefore, there should be no judgment by the United States Supreme Court to reverse the *Roe v. Wade* case—a decision based at that time on the 14th Amendment to the Constitution.

The First Amendment to the Constitution states, "Congress shall make no law respecting an establishment of religion or prohibiting the free exercise thereof; or abridging the freedom of speech, or of the press; or the right of the people peaceably to assemble, and to petition the Government for a redress of grievances."

I would state that it is the First Amendment that protects the woman's right to choose abortion when needed.

Article IV Section 2 of the Constitution states: "The Citizens of each State shall be entitled to all Privileges and Immunities of Citizens in the several States."

The 9th Amendment to the Constitution states: "The enumeration in the Constitution, of certain rights, shall not be construed to deny or disparage others retained by the people."

If abortion were to be made illegal in one or more states, or significant restrictions placed on obtaining an abortion during the first and second trimesters (prior to viability) in one or more states, this would be stating:

- Some religions are preferred over others.
- The citizens in some states do not have the same privileges as a state that allows abortions prior to the point of fetal viability.
- There is not a right to privacy or a right for a woman to decide what health care is appropriate for her own body.

Such decisions would effectively mean that we do not have freedom of religion or the right to privacy in the United States of America.

What do you think our country should do?

Chapter 18: It Has Happened!

But do they have the right to tell the rest of the population what is right?

I receive a daily email from the American Medical Association that reviews news affecting medicine. It is called AMA Morning Rounds. The following is copied from this email on the morning of September 2, 2021:

Leading the News...Supreme Court refuses to block Texas law SB8 prohibiting access to reproductive care

The "New York Times" (9/1, A1, Liptak, Tavernise, Goodman) reports, "The Supreme Court refused just before midnight on Wednesday to block a Texas law prohibiting most abortions, less than a day after it took effect and became the most restrictive abortion measure in the nation." The court's "vote was 5 to 4, with Chief Justice John G. Roberts Jr. joining" in the dissent.

The "Washington Post" (9/1, Barnes, Marimow, Wax-Thibodeaux, Kitchener) reports, "Because the court did not act earlier in the day, the law already had taken effect, and clinics in Texas said they had stopped providing abortions starting at six weeks after a woman's last period." The ban "relies on private citizens to sue people who help women" seeking access to clinical care.

The "AP" (9/1, Sherman, Gresko, Weber) reports that "the American Medical Association said it was deeply disturbed by 'this egregious law' and disappointed by the Supreme Court's inaction. The law 'not only bans virtually all abortions in the state, but it interferes in the patient-physician relationship and places bounties on physicians and health care workers simply for delivering care,' said a statement from" AMA President Gerald E. Harmon, M.D.

On September 9, 2021, the Department of Justice sued the state of Texas over its new law regarding abortion restrictions according to Attorney General Merrick Garland. The lawsuit was filed in federal district court in Austin, Texas. Garland stated, "This kind of scheme to nullify the Constitution of the United States is one that all Americans, whatever their politics or party, should fear" (26).

Even if a woman has regular periods, this does not allow time for detection of pregnancy, consideration for that woman to talk with her doctor and her loved ones about what she thinks is best for her to do—and then schedule a procedure or get medication if she should decide to pursue abortion. The Texas law effectively says that my religion is not acceptable. You would think that the U.S. Supreme Court would not allow such a law to be put into effect given the precedence of *Roe v. Wade*— and the almost 50 years of cases decided since then, while the legal challenges to that law continue through our legal process. But by a vote of 5 to 4, the Supreme Court did allow that law to go into effect. The court at this time is effectively saying it only supports the religion or religions that say that abortion is wrong.

I told you earlier that I respect the belief of people who believe that abortion is wrong— and these people certainly have the right to not have abortions themselves. But do they have the right to tell the rest of the population what is right? Do they have the right to tell the rest of the population what is the correct religion?

In my faith, God does not agree with any of the above, which does not mean that all women who have an unplanned pregnancy should get an abortion. It simply means that each woman can and should decide with her physician and family what is best for her to do.

The Supreme Court might say that I lack "standing" to pursue this issue in the courts. But whether I am male or female, pregnant or not, a physician or some other occupation, the decisions of the Supreme Court have affected my life—but more importantly the lives of millions of women.

Too many women in our country do not have practical access to contraception, whether it is because they are unemployed and lack insurance, or whether their employer believes it is wrong to fund contraception, or whether their employer is a religious organization that happens to not believe in contraception. Too many women in our country with an unintended pregnancy who believe that abortion is an acceptable option—and who do not wish to carry their pregnancy to term—do not have practical access to abortion. The political lobbying arm of the "pro-life" movement has been successful in taking away reproductive rights and privacy rights and freedom of religion rights in many states of our country as well as the country as a whole. Even if the Supreme Court did not further restrict or overturn *Roe v. Wade*, we do not currently have freedom of religion in our country when it comes to reproductive rights.

Also, when you look at the very different levels of access to reproductive health care and policies against abortion in multiple states in our country, the women of our country do not have equal protection under the law.

I must hope and pray that enough citizens of our country act to restore freedom of religion and to protect the rights of women to control what happens to their bodies. In any event, we should make sure that all people have access to whatever method of contraception works best for everyone. We should make sure that all women who have an intended pregnancy have access to high-quality prenatal and postnatal care. We should be doing all that we can to reduce maternal mortality in our country.

But in order to reduce the number of women that die from pregnancy in our country, it is appropriate to have safe and legal abortion available to anyone who believes that is the best option for them to pursue. Remember the medical facts: abortion is safer for a woman than carrying a pregnancy to childbirth.

We still have a very patriarchal society. It has been over 100 years since women earned the right to vote.

✓ Will it take another 100 years for women to have the right to decide what happens to their body without interference from the government or the rest of society?

✓ Will it take another 100 years to not have the threat of intimidation should a woman choose to go to an abortion clinic?

I used to sing in a men's octet in my church. We sang a song called "Find Us Faithful." The lyrics described how being faithful could light the way for others to see—how our lives can inspire others to pursue God and the path God hopes for us to take.

I must hope and pray that God does desire for me to share the thoughts expressed in this book. Again, I respect the people that believe differently than I do. But I also must share my love and concern for all the people of this nation and this world. To me, those Christians who are strongly "pro-life" do not seem to know the love and grace of God. I believe they are stuck in the past, believing in a God who manifested with "fire and brimstone." The God of love and grace would ask each one of us to be with and support the woman who has an unintended pregnancy.

I believe God asks us to support whatever decision the woman makes about whether to remain pregnant or to have an abortion—and God asks us to be *pro-choice/pro-life.*

What should I do?
I trust that each woman, along with her physician and family, can best answer that question.

Acknowledgments

First, I must thank Libby for her encouragement and support, as well as her feedback as I have pursued writing this book. Her belief that it was a worthwhile project and her feedback both as an avid reader, a physician, a woman, and a mother, have given me valuable input. I want to thank my children Chris, Tom, and Sarah and their spouses Julie, Darcy, and Jake for their unwavering support of me. I write because I hope to have some small amount of positive influence on the future that my grandchildren will experience. I want to thank my sister Janet, who helped me both with this book as well as my first book, *I Got to Live With an Angel*. I also want to thank Rolf Olson, who is a pastor in the ELCA, for his foreword. I heard a number of his sermons when he was senior pastor at Richfield Lutheran and have always appreciated the way that he shares the love and grace that God has for us.

Thanks to Connie Anderson (WordsandDeedsInc.com) who did invaluable editing for me, as well as Ann Aubitz, my publisher from Kirk House Publishers, who designed the cover and gave other valuable suggestions.

I want to thank all my friends and extended family members who have helped me to experience God's love and forgiveness. I wish to thank God for my life and all of life.

And finally, I want to thank all women for their part in making this planet a better place, and for making it possible for the human race to continue. Whether each one of you wants to have a pregnancy and child or not, whatever the goals you have for your life, I will pray that you are able to be happy and healthy and can obtain the health care that you desire to have. You have the right to decide what you think is best to happen to you and your body.

Over the course of human history, we men have had plenty of opportunity to affect the course of that history. It is time that we truly embrace the equal role that men and women should play in the future of our species. Together we can make a difference!

References

1. Roosa Tikkanen et al., "Maternal Mortality and Maternal Care in the United States Compared to 10 Other Developed Countries," *Commonwealth Fund* (November 2020). doi:10.26099/411v-9255. Used with permission.

2. Paola Devis and M. Grace Knutlinen, "Deep Venous Thrombosis in Pregnancy: Incidence, Pathogenesis, and Endovascular Management." *Cardiovascular Diagnosis and Therapy* 7, sup. 3 (December 2017): S309–S319. doi:10.21037/cdt.2017.10.08

3. Elizabeth Raymond and David Grimes, "The Comparative Safety of Legal Induced Abortion and Childbirth in the United States," *Obstetrics & Gynecology* 119, no. 2, pt. 1 (February 2012): 215-9. doi:10.1097/AOG.0b013e31823fe923.

4. Katherine Kortsmit et al., "Abortion Surveillance
    — United States, 2018," CDC (November 2020).
    https://www.cdc.gov/mmwr/vol-
    umes/69/ss/ss6907a1.htm

5. Suzanne Zane et al., "Abortion-Related Mortality in
    the United States," *Obstetrics & Gynecology* 126,
    no. 2 (August 2015). https://jour-
    nals.lww.com/greenjour-
    nal/Fulltext/2015/08000/Abortion_Related_Mortal-
    ity_in_the_United_States_.6.aspx

6. Jonathan Bearak et al., "Unintended Pregnancy and
    Abortion by Income, Region, and the Legal Status
    of Abortion: Estimates from a Comprehensive
    Model for 1990–2019." *Lancet Global Health* 8,
    no. 9 (September 2020): e1152-e1161.
    doi:10.1016/S2214-109X (20)30315-6. Used with
    permission from Elsevier.

7. Bela Ganatra et al., "Global, Regional, and Subre-
    gional Classification of Abortions by Safety, 2010–
    14: Estimates from a Bayesian Hierarchical
    Model," *Lancet* 390, no. 10110 (November 2017):
    2372-81.

8. Lisa Haddad, "Unsafe Abortion: Unnecessary Ma-
    ternal Mortality," *Obstetrics & Gynecology* 2, no. 2
    (Spring 2009): 122–26.

9. James Trussell et al., "Efficacy, Safety, and Per-
    sonal Considerations." In *Contraceptive*

Technology (21st ed.). New York, NY: Ayer Company Publishers, Inc., 2018. Used with permission.

10. Audiey Kao, "History of Oral Contraception," AMA Journal of Ethics (June 2020). https://journalofethics.ama-assn.org/article/history-oral-contraception/2000-06

11. Nathalie Kapp and Patricia A. Lohr, "Modern Methods to Induce Abortion: Safety, Efficacy and Choice," *Best Practice & Research Clinical Obstetrics & Gynecology* 63 (February 2020): 37-44.

12. R. Kulier et al., "Medical Methods for First Trimester Abortion," *Cochrane Database of Systematic Reviews* 11 (2011): CD002855.

13. Melissa Chen and Mitchell Creinin, "Mifepristone with Buccal Misoprostol for Medical Abortion: A Systematic Review," *Obstetrics & Gynecology* 126, no. 1 (July 2015): 12-21.

14. Roe v. Wade. www.oyez.org/cases/1971/70-18. Accessed 28 Oct. 2021.

15. "Abortion," Evangelical Lutheran Church in America. https://www.elca.org/Faith/Faith-and-Society/Social-Statements/Abortion

16. Ed Pilkington. "For Years Anti-Abortionists Tried to Stop Doctor Tiller. Finally a Bullet Did," *The Guardian* (June 1, 2009). London. Archived from the original on June 11, 2009. Retrieved Sept. 17, 2021.

17. Mireille Jacobson and Heather Royer, "Aftershocks: The Impact of Clinic Violence on Abortion Services," *American Economic Journal: Applied Economics* 3 (January 2011):189-223. http://www.aeaweb.org/articles.php?doi=10.1257/app.3.1.189. Used with permission.

18. "World Population," Worldometers. https://worldometers.info/world-population

19. Julie Rovner, "Abortion Funding Ban Has Evolved Over the Years," *NPR* (December 15, 2009). Retrieved Sept. 25, 2021. Used with permission.

20. *Harris v. McCrae*, no. 79-1268. Argued April 21, 1980. Decided June 30, 1980.

21. David Blumenthal, Melinda Abrams, and Rachel Nuzum, "The Affordable Care Act at 5 Years." *New England Journal of Medicine* 372, no. 25 (June 2015): 2451–58.

22. Erica Turret, Katherine Kraschel, and Gregory Curfman, "A Further Weakening of Contraceptive Coverage Under the Affordable Care Act," *JAMA Internal Medicine* 180, no. 11 (2020):1415-16. doi:10.1001/jamainternmed.2020.5533

23. Burwell v. Hobby Lobby Stores.
https://www.oyez.org/cases/2013/13-354

24. Lisa Haddad and Nawal Nour, "Unsafe Abortion: Unnecessary Maternal Mortality," *Obstetrics & Gynecology* 2, no. 2 (Spring 2009): 122–26.

25. Susheela Singh et al. "Abortion Worldwide 2017: Uneven Progress and Unequal Access," Guttmacher Institute. Published March 2018.

26. "Attorney General Merrick B. Garland Delivers Remarks Announcing Lawsuit Against the State of Texas to Stop Unconstitutional Senate Bill 8." https://www.justice.gov/opa/speech/attorney-general-merrick-b-garland-delivers-remarks-announcing-lawsuit-against-state-0